THE pH MIRACLE
FOR WEIGHT LOSS

THE pH MIRACLE FOR WEIGHT LOSS

Balance Your Body Chemistry,
Achieve Your Ideal Weight

Robert O. Young, PhD,
and Shelley Redford Young

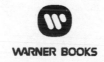

WARNER BOOKS

NEW YORK   BOSTON

Photos on page 19 taken by Kathryn A. Godden and Scott A. Johnson.
Photos on page 42 by James Ward.
"After" photo on page 199 © The Picture People.

Warner Books

Time Warner Book Group
1271 Avenue of the Americas, New York, NY 10020
Visit our Web site at www.twbookmark.com.

Printed in the United States of America

First Printing: May 2005
10 9 8 7 6 5 4 3 2 1

Library of Congress Cataloging-in-Publication Data

Young, Robert O.
    The pH miracle for weight loss : balance your body chemistry, achieve your ideal weight / Robert
O. Young and Shelley Redford Young.— 1st ed.
        p.   cm.
    Includes bibliographical references and index.
    ISBN 0-446-57722-7
    1. Reducing diets.   2. Acid-base imbalances—Complications.   I. Young, Shelley Redford.
II. Title.
    RM222.2.Y684 2005
    613.7—dc22   2004027909

Book design by Giorgetta Bell McRee
Text illustrations by Emma Vokurka

Dedication

"At the center of the universe is a loving heart that continues to beat and that wants the best for every person. Anything we can do to help foster the intellect and spirit and emotional growth of our fellow human beings, that is our job. Those of us who have this particular vision must continue against all odds. Life is for service."

These are the profound and loving words of the late Fred Rogers who taught many of us growing up to serve and love others. As we reflect on the words of Mr. Rogers we must express that our greatest happiness and joy has come when we are in the service of our God, our family, our friends, and our brothers and sisters around the world. We, too, believe that life is for service—life is about changing lives for the better and saving lives from physical, emotional, and spiritual bondage. This is our mission statement and our hope for a better, more righteous and loving world to live in. This is what Jesus taught when he walked the earth—to love and serve God with all our hearts, might, minds, and strength and to love and serve one another.

With love and service as the keystone of our life, it is our honor, privilege, and blessing to dedicate this book first to our God, who has given us life and the reasons to serve; second to our children, Adam, Ashley, Andrew, and Alex, our son-in-law Matthew, and our grandchild CharLee, who teach us through their kindness, love, and example; third to our friend Mr. Rogers and his great example of service to children of all ages; and finally to those children and adults who have felt the pain, despair, and hopelessness of obesity. May this book be an olive leaf of hope and healing.

May our service begin first with selfless acts of love for others and then, and only then, our physical, emotional, and spiritual healing begin to take place in us, followed by healing in our families, next in our communities, then in our nations, and finally in our world.

Acknowledgments

I believe Shelley and I have outlined specific spiritual truths in *The pH Miracle for Weight Loss* that can and will determine the quality and the quantity of your life and set you truly free to live with faith, hope, joy, happiness, love, energy, and passion—free from excess weight, sickness, and disease. We have not completed this work alone or in isolation but with the help of many others who have contributed time and talents in making *The pH Miracle for Weight Loss* a reality.

First and foremost we give thanks and gratitude to a loving Heavenly Father who has blessed Shelley and me with further light and knowledge of spiritual principles or truths to share with our family, friends, and other brothers and sisters of the world to improve the quality and quantity of each individual life on this planet, including all animals and plant life.

To our incredible children, Adam, Ashley, Andrew, and Alex, we give thanks, gratitude, and love for always being supportive in our endeavors of service to others while sacrificing time away from home and from them.

Once again, we must give thanks and gratitude for the life and work of the greatest scientist of the nineteenth century, Antoine Bechamp, and the truths he shared with the world in his final book, *The Blood: The Third Anatomical Element*. His life and work have been a refreshing confirmation that Shelley and I are on the path of truth and light, which leads to the tree of life that has been shown to improve the quality and quantity of life for thousands of folks worldwide.

Our thanks and gratitude to our great, great grandfather, Brigham Young, who taught us the nature of matter from his own words more than one hundred years ago when he said, "Matter cannot be created nor can it be destroyed, it can only be organized or disorganized." With this foundational understanding of matter I was able to view and then document the biological transformation of matter from one form to another form, such as a red blood cell biologically transforming into a bacterial or yeast cell or vice versa.

To our publisher, Warner Books, and especially our editor there, Diana Baroni: our heartfelt thanks and gratitude for having the faith and courage in Shelley and me to publish not just another book on weight loss but the foundational, temporal, and spiritual truths of healthy and long-lasting weight loss free of all sickness and disease.

Our thanks also to our editor Colleen Kapklein, who continues to carefully and thoughtfully weave our words into a beautiful manuscript so that anyone can understand and implement these principles in their daily lives.

To our agents, Richard Hill and Greg Link, we express our thanks for their confidence in and commitment to getting our message out there in the world so that all our brothers and sisters may enjoy the benefits of pH Miracle Living.

To our good and faithful friend and fellow servant Glen Ezekiel, who has always been there to help in all ways—we thank you from the bottom of our hearts.

We express our gratitude and thanks to Jason Moore and Corrine Brandi, who have assisted us in compiling some of the most compelling blood research contained in this book, helping us document the reality of biological transformation and the way life and death begins and ends in the blood with the primary cell, the erythrocyte. In the words of Roman emperor Marcus Aurelius Antoninus, "Nothing has such power to broaden the mind as the ability to investigate systematically and truly all that comes under thy observation in life." We are eternally grateful for your selfless service and commitment to Shelley and me and your fellow inhabitants around the world seeking a better way of living, eating, and thinking.

To the thousands of overweight, underweight, sick, and tired folks worldwide and especially those individuals who demonstrated the faith, hope, courage, and commitment to apply the pH Miracle Living plan of health, energy, and fitness and to make the necessary lifestyle and dietary changes as presented in this book in order to bring about renewed health and energy, a return to a healthy ideal weight, and a renewed passion for life free of all sickness and disease—we are truly thankful. You are an inspiration and a motivation to all who will read your stories of patience, persistence, faith, hope, and commitment. Through your stories, and with the knowledge that *no one* needs to choose to be fat, sick, or tired, lives will be changed for the better and lives will be saved. You have taught us all that being sick, tired, and fat is a conscious choice, not a disease, just as incredible outstanding health, energy, and vitality is something you do, not something you get. Thank you for being shining examples of pH Miracle Living.

Much appreciation goes to the many talented chefs who entered our second pH Miracle recipe contest. Many of your creative and tasty dishes are now at our fingertips because of your generous caring hearts. Thank you for sharing your culinary masterpieces so that all can enjoy and benefit! We'd also like to thank our staff at The pH Miracle Living Center, namely Brock, Matthew, Richard, Edna, Donna, Ashley, and Katie, for preparing, testing, and deciding the winners for the contest. Special thanks to Ashley Young Lisonbee and Donna Downing for their efforts in creating new recipes and preparing all the recipes for publication.

In gratitude, thanks, love, and light,

Dr. Robert and Shelley Young

Contents

Chapter 1

Fat Food Nation

*For new ideas to be accepted, one has to wait for a generation of
scientists to die off and a new one to replace it.*
—MAX PLANCK, 1918 Nobel Laureate in physics

Let's start with a little math. How many pounds do you need to shed
before you reach your ideal, healthy weight? 10? 30? 100?

Whatever your answer, multiply it by 2.

You are now looking at the maximum number of days it will take
you to reach that ideal weight, if you follow the pH Miracle Living
plan. That's right, if your spare tire weighs 15 pounds, you'll be rid of
it in one month—and maybe even in half that amount of time.
Ninety extra pounds weighing you down? Gone forever in six
months—and just as likely in only three. Not just a diet, this is a
complete lifestyle plan. And it works. It has never failed those who
apply its principles. Thousands and thousands of people have
slimmed down to their ideal weights on this plan, dropping an average of a half to 1 pound *each and every day*—and then stayed there.
We are here to tell you: You can, too.

Thought that 90-pounds-in-90-days stuff would get your attention. After all, you're here because, like about two-thirds of Americans—120 million people—you are carrying around excess weight
you want to get rid of. You're part of the 45 percent of American

women and 30 percent of American men who are, at any given moment in time, actively trying to lose weight. We are in the midst of an already staggering—yet still rapidly increasing—worldwide epidemic of obesity. But it is America that is the fattest nation on earth. And we are fatter than we've ever been before—the statistics don't lie.

Nearly one in three American adults is overweight, up from roughly one in four just ten years ago. Nearly half of overweight Americans are officially obese—more than 20 percent above their ideal body weight, or approximately 30 or more pounds over what would be healthy. A study conducted by American Sports Data showed that one in nine adult American men weighs more than 250 pounds, while one in six adult American women weighs 200 pounds or more. The rate of obesity more than doubled between 1960 and 2000, according to the National Institutes of Health (NIH), with a large portion of the increase occurring in the 1990s. By 2040, virtually all of us will be overweight or obese if we don't change our ways. This problem is only going to continue to expand. For instance, 15 percent of American children are overweight or obese. That's nine million children, and another seven million are "at risk"—up from 5 percent of kids in 1980 to these record levels. Overweight children are even more likely to be overweight as adults than their normal-weight peers. The Centers for Disease Control (CDC) reports on research that indicates overweight teens stand an 80 percent chance of becoming overweight adults.

Obesity has risen to be the second biggest cause of preventable death in this country, according to the CDC. Deaths linked to being overweight outnumber those from alcohol, drugs, firearms, and motor vehicles—combined.

In 2003, obesity-related medical costs totaled $75 billion. As you grow fatter, your chance of developing heart disease, diabetes, diabetic complications, arthritis, gallstones, kidney failure, high blood pressure, stroke, and certain cancers, among other deadly conditions, also increases. Even those who aren't overweight themselves have a vested interest in putting an end to this epidemic: Taxpayers cough up roughly $39 billion each year—that's about $175 each—to pay for obesity-related health care through Medicare and Medicaid programs, according to a study co-sponsored by the CDC.

Why the growing epidemic? It could be the barrage of conflicting advice we receive on nutrition from TV, books, and the media. It could be the lack of advice we receive from physicians. A 2000 study released by the CDC revealed that only about 40 percent of doctors advise their overweight patients to lose weight. That's actually a decrease from 1994, despite the fact that this country is fatter now than it was then—and that patients who are counseled by their doctors to lose weight are nearly three times as likely to actually do so than those who don't hear from their doctors on the subject. Maybe a doctor's silence is not so surprising, given how little training most doctors receive in nutrition—and how inadequate is that little training.

Or maybe it is because they simply don't recognize obesity when they see it. Or, at least don't bring it up with patients when they do. A study done in Baltimore and published in 2002 in the *American Journal of Medicine* showed that up to a fourth of doctors didn't take note of their patients' weight problems. (The patients themselves weren't exactly models of perception on this point either—21 per cent of overweight patients believed their weight was normal, and 22 percent of those patients were actually obese.)

It's unclear how much being tuned in to the problem would help, however, because most of what medical science has prescribed to fight fat has had little success over the long haul. We've been told for years and years to eat less and move more, yet still obesity rates have tripled.

Your choice here is to either shake your head at how the medical system has failed us—or you can realize you must take responsibility for your own weight and health. Congratulations; by reading this book you are walking through door number two. You may be surprised by what you'll find there.

America is fatter than it has ever been, and getting fatter every year, because we've been guided, thus far, by a fundamental misunderstanding of how and why the body stores fat. We've focused on false clues and dead ends. The real causes of this plague are largely ignored. This book remedies that, then provides a simple program to allow readers to solve their own personal epidemic of excess weight.

THE IMPORTANCE OF BEING ALKALINE

In this book, I (Rob) put forth the radical proposition that what matters most is keeping your body alkaline, rather than acidic—and how striking that balance allows your body to let go of unnecessary fat cells forever.

Practically speaking, getting to—and keeping—your ideal weight requires eating plenty of high-quality, healthful fats and focusing your food choices around green vegetables. The biggest secret of all is actually in what you *drink,* and this book reveals how keeping your body sufficiently hydrated with the right water makes all the difference. These are the tenets of *The pH Miracle for Weight Loss,* which you won't find anywhere else. This book lays out a simple seven-step plan detailing exactly how you can reach your ideal weight the pH Miracle way.

In this book I also lay out for the first time a specific pH Miracle Living exercise plan to perfectly complement the dietary changes you are making. It totally refocuses the usual emphasis on calorie burning in favor of the single thing that is truly important to weight loss: the right pH balance. Also for the first time, in this book my wife (and coauthor), Shelley, provides menu plans to guide your weight loss, along with her usual heaping helping of brand-new recipes.

Building upon the theory set forth in *The pH Miracle,* which showed how acid/alkaline balance affects myriad health concerns, this book focuses specifically on weight loss. As anyone who has struggled with his or her weight can tell you, finding a healthy, permanent solution to excess pounds is truly miraculous.

Perhaps you've experienced for yourself the failures of some of the nutrition advice currently available. Maybe you're one of the millions of people who have already tried Atkins, The Zone, Weight Watchers, South Beach, or any of the other dozens of programs crowding bookstore shelves and strip malls. If so, you are no doubt familiar with some of the limitations of these programs. Chapter 4 will delve into why each of the popular diets ultimately won't work. Even in the best-case scenario—you actually lose weight—odds are you are going to gain it right back—and then some—because you've dealt with only a symptom and not the underlying cause. Even if you keep the weight off, your victory is illusory: You may be thinner, but you probably won't be healthy.

PROVEN RESULTS

There's a better way. Thousands of people around the world are already walking, talking testaments to the power of this program—living, breathing pH Miracles. I've been watching these amazing results for the past fifteen years. However, once I decided to share the secrets of their successes in a book, I wanted to quantify the results through a controlled study, and I'll present the details of the outcome of my study in a moment. For now, you should know that the twenty-seven participants lost 1,350 pounds—an average of 50 pounds apiece—while decreasing body fat and increasing muscle mass, over just twelve weeks. They lost an average of over a half a pound a day, every day; nearly 15 percent of participants lost a pound a day or more.

Plenty of people with tremendous amounts of weight to lose slimmed down, but they weren't the only ones to benefit. This program also helped individuals get rid of just 10 to 15 unwanted pounds. You'll also hear stories throughout the book of other men and women who have lost weight on the pH Miracle Living plan as well as the many benefits they felt. From them you'll hear the reality behind the theory—real people with real success stories about decreasing blood pressure, cholesterol, and blood sugar levels, and even reversals of established diseases as they reached their ideal weight. The book also includes many dramatic "before and after" pictures worth a thousand words about how this program can transform your life.

Take Sharlene, for example. As with all the terrific men and

women I've worked with whose stories appear in this book, I let you
hear it from her in her own words:

*When the needle on my scale crept up past 300 pounds, I
jumped off and refused to weigh myself anymore. Or to really ac-
knowledge just how heavy I'd gotten. I realize now that I never allowed my picture to be taken while I was at my heaviest. My entire
adult life, my average weight was, I estimate, 274 pounds. Going
over 300 was just too much for me to bear.*

*I've tried just about every diet there is, seems like, including
Atkins, South Beach, The Zone, Eat Right for Your (Blood) Type,
Weight Watchers, Carbohydrate Addicts, and more. I'd tried making bets with friends about who could lose 30 pounds the fastest
(someone else took home the $100). I'd even been almost vegan—
could I have been the world's only fat vegan? I realize, looking
back, that pretty much all I ate were carbohydrates. Since I wasn't
eating meat or dairy or eggs I filled up on pasta, potatoes, and rice.
I packed away twice as much food as my husband and still felt hungry and hollow all the time. I thought I was protein starved.*

I'd lost a hundred pounds twice *before in my life, but I always
felt sick and tired and ended up putting the weight right back on—
and then some. I know now that I was using those diets as temporary fixes and that what is required for permanent weight loss is
permanent lifestyle change. One useful thing I did learn from
Weight Watchers: You have to "live-it" not "DIE-it."*

*My (final!) weight-loss journey began when I joined a Weight
Watchers program at work. With the weekly meetings and weigh-
ins for accountability and support, I started to lose weight. But not
fast enough for me. Until I ran across the pH Miracle program
and decided to give it a try. I actually combined its principles with
the Weight Watchers points system—and finally began losing
weight, and losing weight fast! I lost over 160 pounds in just six
months!*

*I feel like a totally new me. I guess I look like one, too. I recently
ran into an old friend whom I had not seen in about five years. I
realized as she extended her hand to shake mine that she didn't
even recognize me! When I pointed out that she already knew*

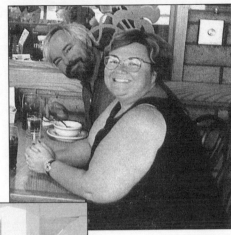

Sharlene before

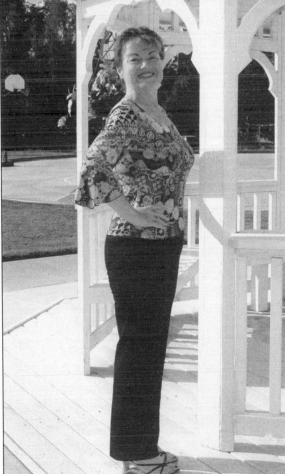

Sharlene after

me—"I'm Sharlene!"—I thought she was going to pass out. My friends say I look younger than ever, and I feel great. I feel more vibrant and alive than I have for the past fifteen years.

Now I'm down to 143 pounds, and the weight is staying off. I've no use for all my size 28 clothes—had to get a whole new wardrobe. In size 6!

Or, David:

Eight months ago, I knew deep down in my soul that I was in trouble. My body was starting to break down and I knew that if I didn't change immediately, I was going to die. I had consumed a plethora of antibiotics over the years. I was using caffeine and sugar to keep me awake and over-the-counter sleeping aids to try to sleep.

Finally, I quit blaming everyone else, including my genes, and decided to take action to change my lifestyle. My goal was not to focus on weight loss. All of my symptoms (acid reflux, prostatitis, hemorrhoids, allergies, depression, heart palpitations, chest pain, and joint pain to name just a few) are found in thin people as well. I saw being overweight as just another symptom of being unhealthy, a visual indicator of my unhealthy lifestyle.

But when I did change, when I focused on optimal health, when I gave up the dream of a magic pill that does it all for you, when I worked the synergy of several approaches at once (drinking my greens, eating well, starting to exercise, thinking good thoughts, helping others)—I lost 100 pounds in eight months. Every single symptom I had is no longer on my health résumé, and I am experiencing a phenomenal quality of life.

In my twelve-week study to quantify the results—which I already knew from experience that this program gets—I followed thirteen women and fourteen men who had tried to lose weight on various popular fad diets. Every person in the study had tried one—or several—popular diets without success and, in some cases, with the creation of symptoms that were worse than simply being overweight, including high blood pressure, high blood sugar, and increased cho-

David before

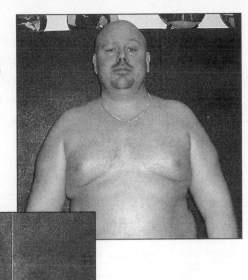

David after

lesterol levels. (They were all getting more and more acidic from diets high in sugars and protein.) No participants had ever reached their ideal weight despite their best efforts.

Participants drank 1 liter of alkaline water (see chapter 5) for every 30 pounds of body weight, every day. They took supplements, including pH drops and powdered greens (in their water, see chapter 9), healthy oils, soy sprouts, and Montmorillonite clay (see chapter 9) as well as an herbal bowel cleanser. And they exercised, at least fifteen minutes a day bouncing on a rebounder (see chapter 10), or thirty minutes a day of walking, swimming, or jogging, five days a week. For those with 50 pounds or less to lose, the first two weeks of the program consisted of a "liquid feast" (see chapter 11), which was extended to three weeks for those with over 50 pounds to lose. Each participant received a 21-day menu plan much like the one in chapter 12 and suggested recipes they could use for meals for the entire twelve weeks. They were advised to eat smaller meals six to nine times a day rather than the conventional three large meals a day.

Every person kept a daily journal of what they ate and drank, what supplements they took, and when and for how long they exercised. And they all had their pictures and measurements taken at the beginning and the end of the twelve weeks as a concrete way of bringing home the results. Both live and dried blood analyses were performed on each person before they began and again after twelve weeks on the program in order to see the difference at the cellular level.

The following chart summarizes the results:

Participant, Age	Beginning Weight (lbs.)	Ending Weight (lbs.)	Total Weight Lost (lbs.)
Male, 52	435	344	90
Male, 48	273	202	71
Male, 45	215	180	35[a]
Male, 34	216	174	42
Male, 46	335	242	93
Male, 42	283	185	98
Male, 48	244	174	70
Male, 29	200	145	55
Male, 58	275	248	27
Male, 53	267	233	34
Male, 52	274	222	52

Male, 61	245	213	32
Male, 48	180	160	20[b]
Male, 36	212	192	20
Female, 58	272	221.5	50.5
Female, 52	158	123	35
Female, 50	140	118	22
Female, 38	200	130	70
Female, 55	340	294	48
Female, 58	160	125	35
Female, 38	265	232	34
Female, 36	210	177	33
Female, 55	307	268	39
Female, 34	180	155	25
Female, 48	225	172.5	52.5
Female, 46	239	148	91
Female, 45	274	202	72[c]

[a] He reached his ideal weight after eight weeks and stayed there; he didn't lose any more weight over the last four weeks.
[b] He reached his ideal weight after four weeks and stayed there; he didn't lose any more weight over the last eight weeks.
[c] She has continued on the program and now weighs 142½ pounds, for a total weight loss of 131½ pounds, which took her from a size 28 to a size 6!

All participants experienced a range of other improvements in their health, including lowered cholesterol, lowered blood pressure, normalized blood sugar levels (and discontinued medications for all three conditions), improved libido, improved muscle tone, and elimination of heartburn, indigestion, constipation, diarrhea, yeast infections, depression, and pain. To name just a few!

PREVENTION AND CURE

The current health care crisis of obesity is entirely preventable, and curable. If we, collectively, drop the pounds, we'll all be healthier and live longer and better. If *you* drop the pounds, *you'll* be healthier and live longer and better. Anyone who has ever struggled with his or her weight knows, however, that it just isn't that simple.

Until now. With this program, it *is* that simple. Follow it, and you will drop those pounds. There's one crucial difference here from everything you've heard before, however. In this book, we're not talking about losing weight in order to get healthy. We're talking about getting healthy first—whereupon your body will let go of the extra weight it has been carrying. Fortunately, even that's simple. The early chapters of this book lay out the basic principles you need to understand in order to succeed, and the remaining chapters give you the practical tools you'll need to do so. Learn them. Use them. And say good-bye to the excess weight you've been carrying around but will no longer need.

Chapter 2

It's Not the Fat, It's the Acidity

Facts do not cease to exist because they are ignored.
—ALDOUS HUXLEY

When it comes to all the extra weight we are carrying around, we have to understand the cause before we can comprehend the cure. Any program that addresses only the obvious symptom of the problem (excess pounds) will never truly solve the problem. It's like pulling a weed without getting the root. To this point, the cause of obesity has been misunderstood anyway. We've been pulling up roots like crazy, but none of them connected to the actual weeds we're trying to rid the garden of! Subsequently, not only do we still have weeds, but also the flowers and plants are suffering.

Weighing too much is *not* about fat. We've been focused on low-fat everything for a couple of decades now, and look where that has gotten us. Nor is it about calories, carbs, or cholesterol. Collectively, we've tried all that, too, and still we, as a nation, are fatter than we've ever been.

That will never change until we grasp what's really at the heart of the matter: acid. The body retains fat as a protection against the overproduction of acids produced by the typical American diet. Some of these acids are eliminated through the bowels, urinary tract, and skin, but whatever is left must be buffered, or neutralized. Excess acid in the body starts to break down cells in your tissues and organs—pretty much the same way acidic steak sauces tenderize meat. Cell breakdown sends the body into self-preservation mode; it uses dietary and body fat in a desperate attempt to protect itself, no matter what the costs. Fat can bind up acids and sometimes escort them out of the body. But fat is used primarily as a way to *store* those acids. Ask any plastic surgeon: The fat they liposuction out of their patients is brown and black because of all the acids it contains. (One of our associates, who is a plastic surgeon, put this to the test by sending samples of liposuctioned fat in for analysis; the lab reports concluded it was indeed full of acid.) In the short term, this is good news: Your body is protecting itself from immediate damage by those acids. The bad news: Over the long term, those fat/acid deposits create a whole bunch of health problems.

The over-acidification of the body sets in motion a destructive cycle of imbalance, overweight, and disease. It's the symptoms we're all looking at, but a cause we are only beginning to understand. Too much acid in the body robs the blood of oxygen, and without oxygen, the metabolism slows. Food digests more slowly, inducing weight gain and sluggishness, and, worse still, causing the food to ferment (rot!). Fermentation creates yeast, fungus, and mold throughout the body. These are all living organisms, so they need to "eat," and when they overgrow in an acidic body they feed on *your* nutrients, reducing the chemical and mechanical absorption of everything you eat by as much as 50 percent. Because they eat, they also produce waste products, and these wastes, called exo*toxins* and myco*toxins,* can be very damaging to your cells. (Our earlier book, *The pH Miracle,* goes into detail about these organisms, along with bacteria, and how they run amok in acidic bodies—and the damage they do.) Without enough nutrients, your body cannot build tissue or produce alkaline buffers, hormones, or hundreds of other chemical components necessary for cell energy and organ activity. In this situation, rather than providing energy, our food remains stagnant in the body and leads to further acidification—a vicious cycle. And the result is unwanted weight gain as well as fatigue and illness.

The bottom line: You are not overweight, you are overacidic.

Your fat is actually saving your life. Without that fat protecting the cells, tissues, and organs of your body from acids, you would be dead. (Similarly, the cholesterol that's long been associated with overweight is also bringing you a benefit: The plaque buildup protects your arteries from acids that could otherwise eat holes right through them.) You should be grateful for your fat! That doesn't mean, however, that you have to want all that fat hanging around. As long as you don't understand why it is piling up, you can't take action to reverse it, and you will actually *need* that fat. With the information here, you'll be able to free yourself from needing that fat. Once you've read through this book, you'll know how to keep acids out of your body in the first place. Then your body can—and will—let go of the excess fat. Simple as that. If your food and drink are alkaline (meaning, in basic chemistry, the opposite of acid), all that acid-binding fat will just melt right off. There will be no need for the body to hold on to it anymore.

UNDERWEIGHT

The majority of Americans who need to lose weight for optimal health may roll their eyes, but a significant number of people also struggle to *put on* weight. The fact of the matter is, underweight and overweight spring from the same source: acidity. The harmful microorganisms that thrive in an acidic environment in your body feed off nutrients that should be nourishing *you*, reducing the chemical and mechanical absorption of everything you eat by as much as half. That alone can cause you to become excessively thin. In addition, underweight people often have damage to a structure in the intestine called the *villus*, and/or congestion from mucus and undigested proteins in the small intestine, both interfering with the assimilation of fats. The body literally wastes away, which can put you at even higher risk of serious illness than an overweight person!

UP YOUR pH

Acidity and alkalinity are measured using the pH scale, as you probably learned back in high school science. Technically, pH is the negative log of the hydrogen ion concentration. In practice, this is a 14-point scale, running from most acidic (0) to most basic (14), with neutral being 7. The farther below 7 you go, the more acidic something is, and the higher above 7, the more alkaline, or basic. pH is a relative, rather than an absolute, measurement; it tells you how acidic or alkaline something is in comparison to something else.

Reaching (and staying at) your ideal body weight is simply a matter of maintaining your body's natural, healthy alkalinity. Anyone who has been living on the typical American diet is most likely going to be too low in pH (too acidic), with a pH level below 7. To achieve healthy and permanent weight loss, my only advice would be to "up your pH!" We'll get to the specifics of how to do that—through the *right* diet, exercise, water, and supplements—in later chapters. Generally speaking, acids and bases (alkaline substances) are opposites and can neutralize each other. But to do so, they have to come together in certain proportions. In the blood it takes about twenty (or more!) times as much base to neutralize any given amount of acid. This means that you need to take in lots more alkaline food than you do acidic food. It also means it is a lot easier to maintain pH balance once you achieve it than it is to get there from an overly acidic state in the first place.

In the same way body temperature is meant to be maintained at 98.6 degrees Fahrenheit, your body is programmed to maintain a pH balance within very narrow parameters. Different areas of the body can have different pH requirements, including some that need to be somewhat acidic, as you can see in the following chart. The best way to determine whether your overall body is in pH balance is by measuring the blood circulating throughout the entire system. Mainstream medicine accepts 7.3 to 7.45 as normal blood pH, with *normal* meaning the usual numbers found in patients. In that case, normal has nothing to do with healthy. By that standard, the normal American is overweight or obese! My research on pH in healthy bodies at healthy weights reveals the desired range to be 7.350 to

7.380—and that ideally it should hit right at 7.365 (slightly alkaline). I consider the medical *normal* to be the range required for survival, whereas ideal represents good health (including healthy weight). Just as with temperature, your pH can vary slightly without causing much concern, but a range too far away from ideal can result in serious consequences.

pH Values for Body Tissue and Fluids

Tissue or Fluid	Standard Normal	pH Miracle Normal (Ideal)
Pancreatic secretions	8.0–8.3	8.2–8.4 (8.3)
Small intestine	7.5–8.0	7.8–9.5 (8.2)
Bile	7.8—8.2	7.8–8.2 (8.2)
Extracellular fluid	7.35–7.45	7.35–7.38 (7.365)
Intracellular fluid	4.5–7.4	7.2–7.45 (7.365)
Venous blood	7.3–7.35	7.35–7.4 (7.365)
Capillary blood	7.35–7.45	7.35–7.45 (7.365)
Arterial blood	7.34–7.45	7.35–7.45 (7.365)
Saliva	6.0–7.0	6.8–7.2 (7.2)
Urine	4.5–8.0	6.8–7.2 (7.2)
Large intestine/colon	5.5–7.0	6.0–7.2 (6.5–7.2)
Stomach	1.0–3.5	3.5–9.5 (5.0–9.5)
Vagina	3.8–4.5	4.0–4.4 (4.2)

Set aside the exact numbers for a moment: Scientists agree that if the body falls out of its delicate pH balance, then vital organs can be damaged and life itself threatened. Therefore, your body will go to great lengths to stay in pH balance—building cholesterol plaques, storing fat, and leaching calcium out of the bones or magnesium out of the heart or muscles to act as buffers—all in an attempt to protect itself from acid damage. None of that is good for your heart, bones, muscles, blood vessels—or waistline!—and puts you on the road to heart attack or stroke, to name just two lurking threats. Bottom line: Balance your pH level by reducing your acidity and you will drop those excess pounds and be on your way to health.

(For a free copy of Dr. Young's article "Acidosis," go to www.pH MiracleLiving.com/bookbonus.)

THE POSITIVE NEGATIVE

The term *pH* derives from German, with *p* standing for "potenz"—power—and *H* being the symbol for hydrogen. Technically speaking, what pH measures is actually the concentration or activity of hydrogen ions in any given solution.

Before we go any further, be forewarned that many of you are about to have bad flashbacks of high school chemistry class. But stick with me for just another minute or two, and I'll make this as simple as I can. Although this program is easy enough to follow even without a more detailed explanation and understanding of pH levels, this background information will make you look at what you eat and drink in a whole new way, a crucial first step on your journey to permanent weight loss. Ready now? Here we go.

An atom is made up of protons, neutrons, and electrons. Protons have a positive charge, electrons have a negative charge, and neutrons have no charge. Atoms always have an equal number of electrons and protons, and the charges cancel out each other. If an atom picks up or loses an electron, it becomes negatively or positively charged, respectively, and becomes known as an ion.

pH measures, in effect, protons and electrons, or positive and negative charges. Below a pH of 7, substances are saturated with protons—hydrogen ions—and are acidic. Above 7, substances are saturated with electrons: alkaline. The more protons, the more acidic. An increase in hydrogen ions (protons) means a drop in pH, and a decrease in hydrogen ions means a rise in pH. Put the other way around, all acids are positively charged, and bases (alkaline things) are negatively charged. Bases can neutralize acids because they have space to accept protons, which their electrons then cancel out.

I'll tell you right now that you are going to have to make a mental note of the fact that what we're after is a negatively charged—alkaline—body. Don't let the usual usage of the words confuse you: When it comes to acid and alkaline, negative is a positive. Alkaline food and drinks, which are negatively charged, bring their life energy into your body.

You need both positive and negative in your body—just like an alkaline battery has a positive and a negative end. To have power and

Laurie

I was very overweight—and very sick. Besides being way too fat, I'd had eight surgeries, and had muscle and nerve damage, thyroid disease, and fibromyalgia. I knew I had to get active, but I hurt all the time. I finally started working out in the water, to

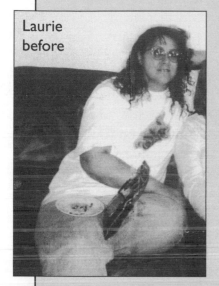

Laurie before

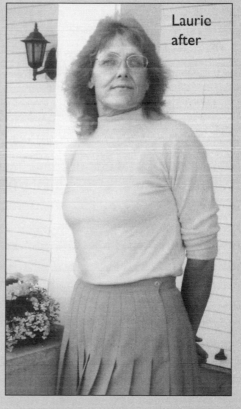

Laurie after

take the strain off my joints and muscles, but even that required a lot of pain medication. Still, I jogged in the pool seven days a week, sometimes for two hours at a time. I was getting stronger—but not losing a pound.

Then, a friend introduced me to the pH Miracle program. She assured me that if I gave the green drink and pH drops at least twelve weeks to do their thing, I would be a whole new person.

I'm here to tell you it didn't take twelve weeks. In barely

three weeks, I felt better than I had in years. I was free of pain! Within twelve weeks, I'd lost 91 pounds (dropping from 239 to 148) and gone from a size 20 to a size 10. It's been a total revolution in my life, and I feel blessed. And healthy.

energy, your body—like the battery—needs to have more electrons than protons. When you take in alkaline—electron-rich—food and drinks, you are in effect recharging your own battery. When you find that negatively charged balance, the body will have no need to desperately soak up and store protons (acids) with fat, and you'll stay at a healthy weight—besides being healthy in general and, quite literally, full of energy.

ARE YOU ACIDIC?

You cannot avoid acid production in your body altogether. Acids are formed during the digestion process (though to a lesser degree on an alkaline diet), respiration, normal metabolism, and cellular breakdown. Before you even account for what happens while you breathe, digestion and metabolism add enough acid to your body to significantly affect its pH, potentially decreasing it by as much as 2 points. That means that unless we help our bodies cope productively with these acid by-products, and/or if we overwhelm the body's ability to do so by piling on acidic food, drink, and behavior, we are destined to remain fat (and sick) (and tired).

Most Americans are caught in the grip of a cycle of imbalance. We eat acidic (proton saturated) foods. We live with negative emotions that, as you'll see in chapter 7, also work against maintaining an alkaline body. Our bodies grow more and more acidic, which causes our healthy cells to change into bacteria, yeast, and molds (as explained fully in *The pH Miracle*). This not only deprives us of healthy cells, but also exposes us to the toxic acidic waste products of these organisms. The body protects itself against the acids as best it

Mike

I'm a forty-seven-year-old EMT and firefighter. I have been overweight most of my life and had little to no energy. I'd come home from work and just hit the couch. But I was tired of friends asking when I was due and all the other fat jokes. I was ready

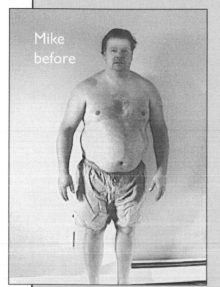

Mike before

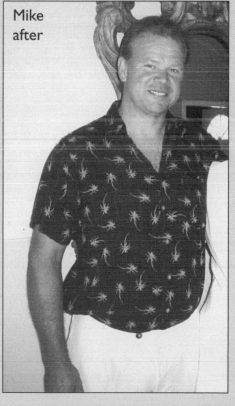

Mike after

to do whatever it took to lose weight.

When I first heard about this program, I took out a calculator and figured I had been alive 2,459 weeks. So trying this plan for twelve weeks was nothing, looking at the big picture, and I decided to go for it. My wife, whose clothes were not fitting anymore and was tired all the time, decided to join me, and we both started with the liquid feast. As my body was cleansed and detoxified, I became aware of how addicted to food I had been. I also saw instant results. Every day I got on the scale, I'd see I'd lost more weight. That really kept me going.

My energy level increased dramatically. I started to wake up earlier to go for walks in the morning. I had so much energy I found myself skipping down the yellow lines in the middle of the road at 5:30 A.M. I was starting to feel young again. My various aches and pains went away.

After two months, I'd lost 50 pounds and my blood pressure came down into the normal range. In less than three months, I'd lost 70 pounds, and my body fat went from 39.4 to 27 percent. I'd lost 12 inches around my stomach and 10 inches off my waist. I'm down to 198 pounds, which I last saw in my teens.

My wife lost 25 pounds and went from a (too tight!) size 12 to an 8, and her energy level increased dramatically too. One day she came home from a bike ride and she just started to cry with happiness, saying she felt like a child again. We are enjoying our alkaline diet together and not missing the old acidic food. People are commenting on how clear our skin and eyes are and how great we look.

I ran into an old friend, and his chin about hit the floor. He said, "I haven't seen you look like this in thirty years!" I went camping with my wife and son recently, and in the morning a friend of my wife's whom I'd only met once before came over to greet us. She apologized for not saying hello the night before, saying, "I saw you over here, but I thought you and Barbara must have split up and she was here with another man!" I thanked her, and agreed. My wife *is* with a new man!

can by binding them up with fat and storing them away. We pile on the extra pounds, feel the aches and pains inevitably associated with acidity, and become vulnerable to sickness and fatigue. Feeling sluggish, we don't exercise. Or we exercise, with the best of intentions, but inadvertently do so in ways that end up making us even more acidic. All this increases our desire for ever more artificial stimulation, whether it be coffee, medications, alcohol, or sugar, making us

Vera

On my sixty-fourth birthday, things didn't look good for my health. I was suffering from several symptoms, including arthritis, low thyroid, acid reflux, and high blood pressure, and between taking all the medication the doctor had prescribed and feeling so lethargic, I had put on 21 pounds. The doctor had told me that, basically, I would have to live with these things, so I had a terrible outlook on life at the time. I had no energy to do normal chores, or even what I love doing most: upholstering furniture.

Finally, I decided that I did not want to live this way and that there had to be something better. The day I started on this program, I put aside all medications and used only green powder and some other supplements—and a whole lot of faith! Within a month, I had lost all the excess weight, all 21 pounds, and all of my symptoms had vanished. I was a bundle of energy once again. Today I am celebrating a wonderful sixty-fifth birthday—feeling better than I did at thirty-five!

more and more acidic. The cycle keeps right on going, picking up momentum with every turn around the track.

Any of that sound familiar? I'm not describing anything unusual; it's just the typical American lifestyle. Just in case you're still not sure this approach is what you need, take a quick look down the following list, counting up 1 point for any item that is currently part of your life. If you total 4 or more points, your body is no doubt acidic, you are most likely overweight, and you are at risk not only for obesity, but also for heart disease, diabetes, stroke, certain kinds of cancer, as well as other health problems. Here's the list:

- fruit or fruit drinks
- alcohol or recreational drugs
- simple carbs, including bread, pasta, potatoes, and baked goods
- cigarettes or other tobacco products
- meat, including chicken, pork products, beef, turkey
- eggs or dairy products
- coffee or tea
- processed food or fast food
- sugar
- soda or sports drinks
- no daily exercise
- stress, negative emotions, or spiritual emptiness

In other words: *This means you.* You can go ahead and get the pH of your blood measured, but I'm confident in saying you're going to discover the number is too low. In fact, you *should* get your pH measured (see chapter 3), because checking it again after four weeks on this program will convince you of the importance of keeping your body alkaline. In case you want more proof than what's showing up on your scale!

[Your doctor can send your blood to a lab to check its pH; it generally takes about four weeks to get results. You can measure the pH of your urine first thing in the morning with special pH paper (available at your local pharmacy, or from The pH Miracle Living Center; see Resources in the back of the book); it should be between 6.8 and 7.2, with 7.2 being ideal. This won't be as revealing as the blood, but it will at least tell you generally whether or not your body is in pH balance.]

You can't escape acids altogether. The body creates them through digestion, metabolism, respiration, and cellular breakdown. What you can do is eliminate the acids you take into your body and consume lots of alkaline food and drink to enable your body to buffer the naturally occurring acids.

A healthy body naturally maintains its own ideal weight. The program laid out in this book is designed to produce that healthy, lean body by nourishing and alkalizing every single cell you have. Restoring balance to your system will create a new level of energy and mental clarity—and allow your body to seek its own ideal weight, naturally.

Chapter 3

What's Blood Got to Do with It?

For the life of all flesh is the blood.
—LEVITICUS 17:14

In a word, everything. Blood's central role in your health and weight makes sense when you consider just how much of it your body contains—exactly how much of your body *is* blood. Everyone has about 5 liters of the stuff. To circulate it through the body, the heart beats over 100,000 times a day, moving two and a half ounces of blood with each pulse—about 8 tons each day. All the blood in the body passes through the heart every three minutes.

You probably already know that red blood cells deliver oxygen throughout your body and remove cellular wastes. Beyond that, even, your blood holds the key to living at an ideal, healthy weight. First of all, the blood dictates your body's internal environment: acidic blood, acidic body; alkaline blood, alkaline body. In addition, your blood cells eventually become body cells (and vice versa). You need to keep your blood clean and pure—and nonacidic. I choose the food and drinks I recommend accordingly: They will build healthy blood cells. Your body makes between 3 and 4 million new blood cells and 11 to 13 million body cells *every second,* so you need to make sure it has the very best materials to work with at any given time.

Later in this chapter, I'll tell you how and why I always put my clients' blood under a microscope—in a procedure different from anything traditional doctors or labs do—and what I can learn from the astonishing things I see. You'll see a series of pictures of real clients' blood samples, taken before and after they followed this program; so you can see for yourself the dramatic difference adhering to these principles makes. But first, let's start with some background on how blood is made and what blood makes, so you can truly understand how crucial healthy blood is to permanent healthy weight loss.

Blood is the most basic material of the human body. Body cells from all types of tissue are continually being formed from the blood. It's actually a two-way street, and body cells can also be transformed into blood cells. Better, however, is when the body follows the normal course of blood production, which is intimately connected to both digestion and respiration. Not only are you in this most fundamental way literally what you eat (and drink), but also what you breathe.

Normal blood cell production originates in the small intestine. Nutrients set free by the digestion process are circulated through the delicate microvilli (microscopic fibers lining the villi of the intestine walls) along the (9 yards of) small intestine, and into the bloodstream, building blood cells, tissues, and organs. Air breathed in through the lungs enters the arteries and chemically unites with the minerals and other elements in the blood to create new blood cells. These red blood cells can then be transformed into bone cells, muscle cells, heart cells, liver cells, and so on, as needed.

When your body is healthy, and you are eating alkaline/electron-rich food, you build healthy blood cells—and so healthy body cells. The digestive process breaks down the foods you eat through a clean, efficient process called oxidation/reduction, which bathes the body cells in a continuous supply of oxygen. Your body stays energetic—and stays at a healthy weight.

When you are subsisting on acidic/proton-rich food, and the intestine becomes damaged or congested, blood production is impaired or stops. In order to keep constant the amount of red blood cells in the body (five million per cubic millimeter!), the body will convert body cells to blood cells—literally wasting away.

As is the blood, so is the body. As is the body, so is the blood. The quality of the blood—and so, the body—depends on the quality of what we eat and drink. If you are eating acidic foods you will have weak blood cells and then weak body cells—and you'll be overweight. You have another choice: With alkaline food and drinks, you'll build healthy blood—and a healthy body, which naturally seeks its own ideal healthy weight (hear an audio of Dr. Young on "Life and Death Is in the Blood" at www.pHMiracleLiving.com/bookbonus).

LIVE BLOOD ANALYSIS

I estimate I've performed blood tests on about ten thousand people in the course of my research over the past twenty years. What I've seen makes a more dramatic case for this program than anything I could tell you in just words. I think you'll agree after you look at the following samples: The blood of a person eating a standard American diet of acidic foods looks incredibly different from the blood of someone eating alkaline. I arrived at the principles of the pH Miracle through observing differences in the blood I tested, and each new set of "before-and-after" blood tests I see confirms their power.

My main techniques differ from those of standard laboratory tests, which can involve fixing blood on a slide with preservatives before putting it under a microscope. Stains may be used to help show up white blood cells, sickle cells or some other distinctive condition, or bacteria, although the addition of those chemicals compromises the blood sample and changes the way it looks. Or the blood drawn in your doctor's office is put in a vial, sent to a lab, spun to separate out the various elements, and weighed with specialized machinery to determine the density of the blood—no microscope needed. In any event, blood prepared in these ways is no longer a living substance. And the purpose of these tests is generally quantitative (i.e., how many white blood cells are there? How many red blood cells?) rather than qualitative (what is the condition of the cells?) like mine. They may also be useful in diagnosis or pathology.

(I do often use standard blood tests as well as my techniques, because there is value in knowing both the quality and the quantity. Results can confirm my observations. I may interpret the results differently than a mainstream physician would, however. In any case, you get the most complete picture by seeing what you can see with all of these approaches.)

I'm more interested in the quality of the blood cells than the number. I take two complementary approaches. The first is live blood analysis. I take a drop of capillary blood from the fingertip, put it on a slide, and place it immediately under a high-powered microscope using the phase contrast setting, which filters and diffuses the light to make transparent objects visible as various shades of gray. I project the image, live, onto a video screen. The point is to see the blood live, right out of the body, and to see the state of the cells and the environment in which they live. All this allows me to see the structure and strength of the red and white blood cells, and the cleanliness of the plasma fluid that surrounds them.

My second technique is dried blood analysis, or what I call the mycotoxic oxidative stress test (MOST). This time blood taken from the fingertip is pressed onto a slide and allowed to air dry. It is then examined under a high-powered microscope, this time using the bright field setting. Most of the light passes directly through the specimen, which shows up details like whether or not the blood is coagulating too much or too little, cellular breakdown, irritation, inflammation, congestion, acidosis, signs of parasites, and even specific organ imbalances. Here I'm looking for certain patterns in the blood drops, especially in regard to aspects of clotting. Under stress of various kinds, the pattern deviates from normal.

The most useful thing about both live and dried blood analyses is that they give you early warning of possible upcoming health issues. Stresses on your body are often observable as abnormalities in the blood long before they manifest as symptoms. You see the genesis of symptoms before they are expressed. These tests are one better than preventive medicine. They are *preemptive* medicine. If you take action to correct what you see, you can save yourself from ever developing the symptoms or conditions you can see first in the blood.

With these blood tests, I am looking, in general, for

- the condition of the red blood cells including size, shape, and symmetry
- the activity level of the immune system (white blood cell activity)
- the presence of blood clots or blood clotting factors
- the presence of parasites, yeast, fungus, bacteria, and/or mold
- the presence of crystalline structures such as arterial plaques, protoplasts, fibrous thallus, uric acid, cholesterol, and crystallized exotoxins and/or mycotoxins
- protein masses indicating cellular breakdown and/or inflammation
- the acidity level and effects of acidity

I can also see signs of specific conditions in the patterns I observe, including

- liver, kidney, pancreatic, heart, lung, prostate, ovarian, breast, and other organ stress
- gastrointestinal tract dysfunction
- degenerative conditions including cancer, diabetes, stroke, high blood pressure, and heart disease
- allergies
- adrenal stress
- poor circulation

In addition, these blood tests can guide your nutritional program. They can be used to identify and monitor your condition and your healing approach. They can reveal

- metabolic dysfunction and blood sugar imbalances
- malabsorption of fats, proteins, vitamins, and other nutrients
- nutritional deficiencies

These final points are the most immediately relevant to the pH Miracle Living plan for healthy weight loss. For one thing, there's no better motivation to make the changes you know you need to make than to get a good, honest look at what exactly is circulating through

Elaine

I've been searching for answers to my weight problem on and off for thirty years. I've tried just about every weight-loss program, including high-protein (and fat!) regimens, without success. I'd all but given up the quest. But this morning I hit the lowest

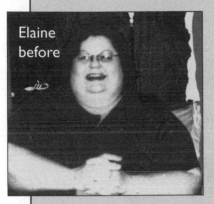

Elaine before

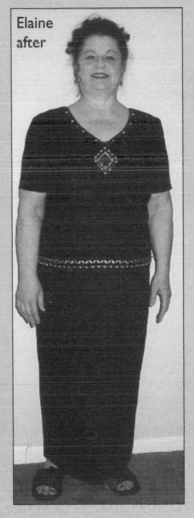

Elaine after

weight I've seen in over twenty years. I lost just over 90 pounds in the first twelve weeks—over half a pound every day! There were 7½ less inches each around my waist, hips, and chest. Three months later, I've lost a total of 77 pounds. I feel light as air knowing my target of 142 pounds will soon be mine.

Never in my wildest dreams did I expect the type of weight loss I've experienced week after week. In fact, as I started this program I wouldn't allow myself to become excited. I'd suffered "the agony of defeat" too many times on other diets.

But I took the leap of faith to try one more time. I committed 100 percent to being totally alkaline and followed the program honestly to the best of my ability. I had at least 5 liters of green drink every day, and sometimes as many as 8 liters. Now I can truly say I'm glad I left those good southern-fried pork chops, biscuits, and gravy far behind me! I'm filled with more determination each day, and my hopes are renewed as the weight keeps coming off.

What's more, I can feel health seeping back inside me. My cholesterol dropped 39 points, well into the healthy range. My blood pressure normalized. My blood sugar is down and I've been able to stop my medication. The age spots on my hands are actually fading! And, jewel beyond price, my singing voice is starting to come back after thirty-one years missing in action.

Overwhelming results like this make it easy to stay focused on my goal. I think not so much of the weight I want to be, but of my thirty-third wedding anniversary next year. I want to have my picture taken for the occasion—wearing my wedding dress. It has been cleaned and waits in the wings. I hung the veil on the wall in my bedroom; it is a reminder of the time I'll be the right size to again wear the dress that goes with it. It *will* happen; I feel it and envision it often. I'll wear that veil proudly, as a crown for a job well done. I'll know I earned it.

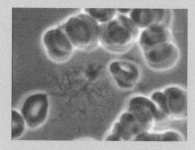 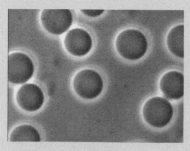

Elaine's blood before   Elaine's blood after

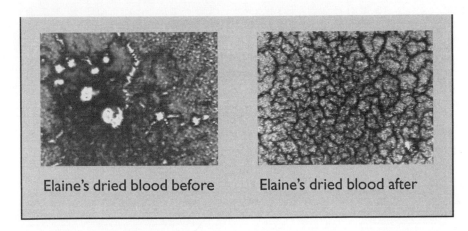

| Elaine's dried blood before | Elaine's dried blood after |

your body—and no better way to commit to those changes permanently than to see, right before your eyes, what an incredible difference they make.

THE PICTURE'S WORTH A THOUSAND WORDS

So, have a look at the picture on the left below, which is a still from a live blood sample, typical of blood with acidic diets and lifestyles. The blood cells are irregularly shaped, and different sizes, and many are sticking together. There are a lot of white blood cells in there trying to clean up the mess. You can see the yeast and the bacteria, as well as aggregations of cellular debris, formations made of crystallized acids, bacterias, yeasts, and molds.

The contrast is obvious with the picture on the right, showing

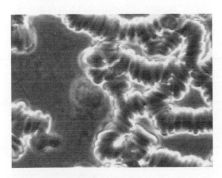

Live blood acidic diet

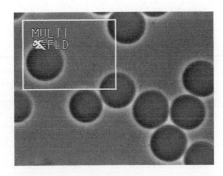

Live blood alkaline

clean, alkaline blood—my blood, in fact. The red blood cells are all the same size, are all nicely round, and are not sticking together. There are no yeasts, molds, bacterias, or white blood cells.

In other words, this is your blood on acid; this is your blood on greens and good fats. Any questions?

Dried blood pictures show an equally dramatic contrast (below). On the acidic blood on the left, you'll see pasty white masses of proteins from cellular breakdown, an abnormal clotting pattern common in diets high in protein or carbohydrate. On the right is a picture of alkaline blood, with normal clots and no polymerization of protein.

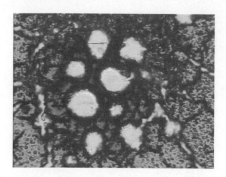
Dried blood acidic diet

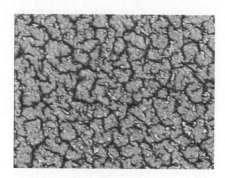
Dried blood alkaline

A BRIEF HISTORY OF BLOOD TESTS

I stand on the shoulders of giants when it comes to carrying on the work of live and dried blood analysis. I am forever indebted to the great scientists who have paved the way for me.

Viewing live blood under a microscope has been around as long as the microscope itself. In the mid-nineteenth and early twentieth centuries, European scientists including Dr. Antoine Bechamp and Dr. Gunther Enderlein proposed new ways of interpreting what was being viewed in the blood. In the late 1800s, Dr. Bechamp documented the changeability of cells, as he witnessed the biological transformation of a red blood cell to a rod bacteria, for example, and other body cells change both their form and their function. (My first book, *The pH Miracle*, contains more detail on this phenomenon, known as pleomorphism.) In the late 1940s, Dr. Enderlein watched the progression go a step further, red blood cell to bacteria to yeast.

By the 1920s, European medical practitioners added another twist when they began looking at dried blood samples. The blood showed similar patterns in patients with similar conditions, revealing characteristic "footprints" of certain pathologies. For instance, in advanced degenerative disease, the blood shows poor clotting, minimal fibrin formation, and many white "puddles" of proteins from cells that have broken down—compared to a tight, fibrin-rich clotting pattern with no white puddles in healthy controls.

The dry blood test made it to America in the 1930s, where it has been handed down from one generation of practitioners to the next outside of the formal channels of medical and biochemical education. Although this test is not done in any commercial lab in the United States, today, hundreds of health care practitioners around the world keep these principles in practice. I'm proud to be one of them.

OMAHA

For the past fifteen years, I've been evaluating the diets and looking at the blood of a group of hundreds of clients in Omaha, Nebraska, going back at least twice each year. I've been seeing many of the same folks for all that time. It's been a learning experience for me as well as them. They get to see what happens to their health—and their blood—as they start applying my principles, and what happens when they go back to a standard American diet. And so do I!

What I've observed has guided me as I prepared the recommendations in this book, helping me to determine the impact of certain foods and supplements on the body at the cellular level. I've been able to watch the impact of different types of diets on the blood, homing in on alkaline, electron-rich greens and polyunsaturated fats as key ingredients in healthy blood, healthy cells, and healthy, ideal-weight bodies. Acidic diets, on the other hand, pollute the blood and compromise cellular structure. As I continued my research, I learned that I could not only tell which blood was acid and which alkaline by looking at it live, but also I could discern patterns in the unhealthy blood that associated with specific health problems. Over and over again, I witnessed what I've come to call the pH Miracle: As acidic patients switched to an alkaline lifestyle, their blood became clean, they lost weight, and they became stronger, more energetic, and healthier.

I've got filing cabinets full of pictures of Omaha blood, but here I'll share just one representative example with you. The changes after this patient followed a program like the one laid out in this book are dramatic. But I've chosen to showcase this client not because her results are extreme, but because they are typical. In other words, this could be you—both the before and the after.

In the next chapter, you'll see even more pictures of the blood, this time taken from people following specific fad diets—then switching to the pH Miracle Living plan. There you'll see even more dramatic differences in before-and-after pictures. Plus, those people were working with a more formatted pH Miracle Living program, as part of a controlled study, for those of you who like to see strict scientific formality before you are convinced.

For now, consider getting an analysis of your own blood. Admittedly, this program is going to take some work on your part, and it requires significant lifestyle changes. I know from experience the amazing motivation that comes from seeing the state of your own blood. It will move you to take action like nothing else ever has. And after twelve weeks, you'll get clear-as-day proof that all you are doing *is* making a difference.

It is critical that you see the inside as well as the outside of your body. If the blood is sick, you will be, too—and fat—regardless of what you look like on the outside. Healthy, permanent weight loss comes from the inside out, starting with clean blood and healthy red blood cells.

Andrea

I was a big skeptic when I went to have my blood tested. But I had struggled so long with my weight, and a number of 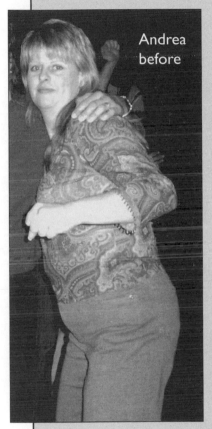 health problems, that anything that promised some relief seemed worth a try. I devised my own little test to see if this really worked: I didn't re-

Andrea before

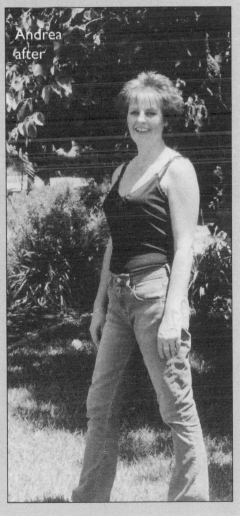

Andrea after

veal anything at all about myself or my health.

Or I should say, I didn't *say* anything about myself in advance. My blood, however, revealed quite a lot on its own.

From live blood analysis, I was informed that I was following a high-protein diet (my blood was full of the acidic wastes thereof), and that I craved sugar and carbs (thanks to all the yeast visible in my blood). The list of likely symptoms associated with the patterns showing in my blood matched just about everything I had been going through.

At the time, I'd been following the Atkins diet, more or less, for six years. My diet consisted of one to two pots of coffee a day, with creamer and artificial sweetener; at least half a liter of diet cola; as well as protein shakes, meat, and dairy. Once in a while, I had junk food. I did get eight to ten glasses of water, at least.

And I thought (at least until I saw my blood) that I was doing pretty good, food-wise! I'd struggled with my weight and body image since I was a child, including bouts with bulimia as well as extreme calorie restriction and self-imposed vomiting that now seem to me like just this side of anorexia. I'd also obsessively exercised, hitting the gym four to five days a week for two hours at a time for a long stretch of my life—which did at least serve to get me down to 135 pounds over the course of nine months. There were also, at various times, laxatives, diet pills, and diet shakes (*gaining* weight, little by little, all the while). A vegetarian phase, with no dairy, helped me lose weight, but this lasted only a few months. There was a period of daily swimming, during which my weight climbed to 185 pounds. I followed a fat-free plan for years, but my body stayed fat nonetheless. Finally, I tried Atkins and was immediately hooked. I lost 50 pounds in less than six months. After a number of years of this, however, my weight started to edge up again, and my health was the pits.

There's something very powerful about seeing your own blood—and everything going on in it—live, right in front of you. I decided then and there that I couldn't go on like that. I have not had a cup of coffee or a soda in the three months since. I've been eating alkaline and drinking greens. I have lost 28 pounds. And my blood now has those even, round circles that mean your body is alkaline—and healthy.

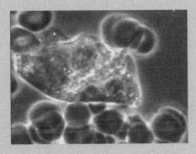
Andrea live blood before

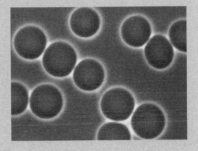
Andrea live blood after

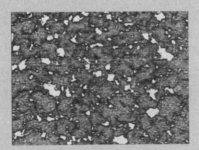
Andrea dried blood before

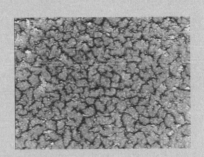
Andrea dried blood after

Chapter 4

Pick a Diet, Any Best-Selling Diet—And I'll Show You Why You're Still Fat (And Sick. And Tired)

Better keep yourself clean and bright;
you are the window through which you must see the world.
—GEORGE BERNARD SHAW

The rising tide of obesity in this country (and around the world) directly correlates with the "low-fat" era of nutrition advice. Paradoxically, trying to avoid fat seems to be making us fatter than ever. The most current antidotes—low-carb, high-protein regimens—may provide temporary results if you are concerned only about the numbers on your scale. They often include more fat in the diet—the toxic, artery-clogging kind. Even without that, the excessive protein dangerously stresses your intestines, kidneys, and liver, and weakens your bones. You might possibly get thinner, temporarily, but you probably won't become any healthier.

Nevertheless, Americans are spending more than $40 billion a year on various diet programs and products, such as Atkins, South Beach, Sugar Busters, Weight Watchers, The Zone, Eat Right for Your (Blood) Type, and so on—and $15 billion a year for low-carb products. Each program offers its own spin on the cause of and solution to overweight and obesity, with its own list of foods to eat and avoid, in what proportions. What all these have in common, with each other and with conventional low-fat/food-pyramid wisdom or conservative Weight Watchers approaches, is that they will make your body moderately to highly acidic. Each and every one recommends foods that can create a pH imbalance in your body, polluting your blood. An imbalance can make you sick—and fat. And keep you fat. In the long run, you will probably regain any weight you did manage to lose, and, in the case of high-protein diets, if you continue it for any length of time (generally over one year), serious sickness or disease may result.

That's right: Following most fad diet plans will, eventually, help you *gain* unwanted weight, as your body desperately protects itself from acidity by piling on the fat. The only true and lasting solution to overweight, I believe, is providing your body with healthy, alkaline blood—something you won't get with anything on the current best-seller lists.

Take for example the latest craze, the South Beach Diet, which recommends a high level of quality, lean protein and moderate levels of fat and carbohydrates. As I see it, the problem with that protein, besides just the vast quantity of it, is that the chicken, turkey, and eggs the author emphasizes are all highly acidic and proton-rich. Reading through the South Beach recipe for Coconut Chicken, for example, I noted a number of moderately alkaline ingredients—the "veggies," which consist of nothing more than onion and scallion; healthy coconut milk, olive oil, and macadamia nuts; and spices measured by the teaspoon, or less. But all that is quite literally outweighed by the chicken and other acidic ingredients, including a sugar substitute. Furthermore, everything is cooked so long that the electron-rich ingredients are compromised, and the otherwise healthful oil may become toxic. Your blood will be thoroughly acidic within minutes after dining on this dish. In my review of Dr. Agatston's menu plans and recipes, I did not find a single recommendation that did not have major or minor ingredients that were acidic. Even if you were to lose weight on this plan, it wouldn't necessarily be a healthy weight loss.

A nutritional analysis of the Atkins diet by the Physicians Committee for Responsible Medicine revealed problems with following that program. Their review showed that the menu plans in all three phases of the Atkins program are consistently high in saturated fat and cholesterol and very low in fiber, and frequently deficient in the seven key vitamins and minerals they measured. The menu plans include, as promised, plenty of protein (between one-quarter and one-third of calories) and very little in the way of carbohydrates (between 3 and 22 percent of calories). You'd also get 45 to 64 percent of your calories from fat, roughly a quarter to a third of that from saturated fats, which raise the risk of heart disease—between 38 and 45 grams each and every day. Fiber tops out at 18 grams in a day, though only in the maintenance phase; before that you'll get an average of a mere 2 to 7 grams a day. Compare that to the 20 to 35 grams generally recommended to lower risk of chronic diseases and control weight. The Atkins menus were also deficient in all of the key nutrients measured: calcium, iron, vitamin C, vitamin A, folate, vitamin B_{12}, and thiamine. (Even the Atkins program itself suggests taking calcium and magnesium supplements.) And that's if you're satisfied to go by the extremely low standards of daily values, which are calculated to prevent diseases of deficiency, not meant to measure how much is required for general good health. Last, but definitely not least, Atkins, like all high-protein diets, is highly acidic, consisting almost entirely of proton-rich foods.

HIGH PROTEIN, HIGH RISK

The Atkins diet is, of course, the longtime leader of a pack of high-protein, low-carb diets, too numerous to list comprehensively. Whatever the specifics of their individual take on the subject, these plans generally have too much protein and unhealthy fat, not enough fiber, and insufficient levels of key vitamins and minerals. And they'll all make your body acidic—and thus, sick, tired, and primed to gain weight.

Research published in the elite medical journals, including the *Journal of the American Medical Association* (*JAMA*) and the *New England Journal of Medicine* (*NEJM*), concludes that following such a high-protein diet for any significant length of time can put you at an increased risk for heart disease and heart attack, kidney disease and kidney stones, diabetes and diabetic complications, certain types

Debra

I was on a popular high-protein diet for about 3 years. I went from 180 to 160 pounds during the first year, but after that I hit a plateau. Eventually, I lost about another 5 pounds. But after 2 years on this diet, I started to notice I had less energy and felt

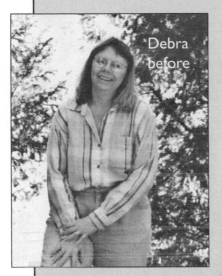

Debra before

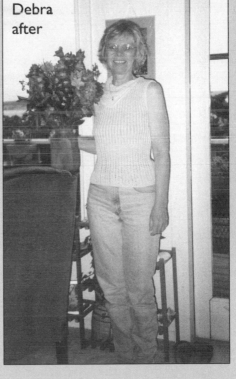

Debra after

weak and light-headed. Sometimes I felt I was close to passing out. I also had migraines. I was losing muscle tone and had chronic pain. And, I started regaining the weight I had worked so hard to lose, even though I wasn't eating any differently than I had been. At the 2½-year mark, I started having alarming changes in my monthly cycle, as well as edema [swelling] in my hands and feet. I developed severe chest pains, and my heart would pound, skip beats, and beat irregularly besides.

Thank God I found a better way. I have spent years researching and experimenting with various diets and "lifestyles," a high-protein diet being just one of them, but it wasn't until the pH Miracle program that I finally felt I had found a wise and effective way of eating and living that truly supports health, fitness, rejuvenation, and a life of balance rather than imbalance. Once I made a commitment to following the pH Miracle plan, hydrating with green drink and eating alkaline foods, I immediately felt better. My energy returned, my headaches vanished, my monthly cycles normalized, my edema disappeared, and my irregular heartbeats stopped. And I began to shed excess acidic fat from my body. All in all I lost 35 pounds, to reach 123.

of cancer (particularly colon cancer), gout, and osteoporosis. Many people restrict their physical activity while on a high-protein/low-carb plan, and the additional risks of lack of exercise are well known. If you can't get worked up about what can happen to you over the long haul, perhaps the potential immediate risks will convince you: mood disturbances, constipation, bad breath—and fatal cardiac arrhythmias. (For a free copy of Shelley Young's article "So . . . What Can I Eat," go to www.pHMiracleLiving.com/bookbonus.)

In addition to the health risks agreed upon by mainstream medical science, my own blood research shows that high-protein diets can interfere with healthy red blood cell production by congesting the bowel and clogging up the villus in the small intestine. With normal red blood cell production stopped, body cells are called upon to be transformed into blood cells in order to keep the required density of blood cells. To my way of thinking, the reason some people lose weight on these diets is that their bodies are literally wasting away, seriously compromising their health in the interest of weight loss that is bound to be temporary anyway.

IF I DON'T DIE, AT LEAST I'LL BE SKINNY

If you've gotten so frustrated with controlling your weight that you are even willing to risk your life and health to shed some pounds, even temporarily, I've got some important news for you: Studies at Duke and the University of Pennsylvania, among others, show that six months on a high-protein, low-carb diet can result in a reduction of about 20 pounds—or, just about exactly the same as the low-fat, moderate-protein diets that are generally regarded as healthy and safe. Research published in *JAMA* that reviewed more than one hundred studies on high-protein/low-carb diets and low-fat/moderate-protein diets concluded that the amount of weight lost correlated with length of time spent on a given diet, and with the number of calories ingested—but not with reducing carbohydrate intake. We shouldn't be surprised: Vegetarians, who generally eat diets rich in carbohydrates, have significantly lower body weights, overall, than people who eat meat. In fact, when switching to a vegetarian diet, most people lose about 10 percent of their body weight.

I'm not, however, recommending a low-fat diet like the government food pyramid, Dean Ornish's program, Weight Watchers, the American Heart Association and American Diabetes Association plans, and the like. You'll get the details on the importance of including plenty of *healthy* fats in your diet in chapter 6. Beyond that, the low-fat diets in studies like the ones I'm talking about here are still full of acidic, proton-rich foods. There's nothing wrong with carbohydrates per se—they are a part of the pH Miracle Living plan—but there are specific types of carbohydrates that will make you acidic. Low-fat diets are, by necessity, high in carbohydrates, but if you're getting acidic carbs (simple carbs your body handles just the same as any sugar), you'll be providing sustenance not only for you but also for the bacteria, yeasts, and molds running rampant in your body. Overwhelming your body with, essentially, sugar this way can lead to sugar intolerance, prediabetes and, eventually, diabetes. It can also stress your adrenals, making you, among other things, tired. And, to protect yourself from acid damage, you'll get fat.

I don't know about you, but for me, any eating plan should not only promote weight loss but also *health*. There are plenty of people apparently willing to live with the health consequences of any plan, as long as it results in short-term weight loss. An eating plan, even a diet, should be nutritious, providing everything the body needs for radiant good health and nothing that will detract from that. Most of what's been available up to now has failed that basic (alkaline!) test. And so ultimately they fail when it comes to permanent weight loss as well. The focus at various times on calories, high-protein, low-fat, low-cholesterol, or a series of other red herrings means we've overlooked the one thing that matters most when it comes to living at your ideal healthy weight: the acidity or alkalinity of what you eat and drink.

Richard

I'd reached the point that when climbing stairs I really thought my heart would stop. I was having all kinds of health problems, including sleep apnea (requiring a breathing machine at night), borderline glaucoma, loss of sensation in my leg and foot, and a bout with a flesh-eating bacteria that put me in the hospital for ten days (without healing—it recurred periodically after that). I weighed 450 pounds, and I knew I had to reduce my weight substantially, and soon, or I was going to die.

I'd tried various diets, both conservative and trendy, but nothing worked well for me until I found this program. With proper foods and nutrients bringing my body into pH balance, I have lost 205 pounds! I feel more energetic than I have in many years; I'm regaining feeling in my leg and foot, my eyesight is clear, there's been no sign of the bacteria, and I have been off my breathing machine for three and a half months now. Why didn't the doctors tell me about this? Having returned to health after years of being sick and tired, I am walking proof that there *is* help out there.

THIS IS YOUR BLOOD ON PROTEIN . . . ANY QUESTIONS?

Every last criticism of the high-protein and high-carb diets shows up in the blood. In fact, those ways of eating have still more flaws that mainstream science has yet to connect the dots on, but they are all clearly expressed in the blood for anyone who wants to look, with live and dried blood analysis. In the following pages, you'll see what the blood of people on these various diets looks like under my microscope, in comparison to that of the same people following the pH Miracle plan. Hint: I've yet to find a person with clean blood on the standard American diet or any of the recent diet crazes.

These amazing before-and-after pictures of my clients' blood samples as they move from fad diets to an alkaline lifestyle make clear the drastic effects on your body of what you eat. They are definitely worth more than a thousand words on why it is important to choose correctly.

This first set of illustrations shows live and dried blood on someone following basically the standard American diet—too much fat (unhealthy fats), too many carbs, not enough vegetables.

1. In live blood analysis of blood from a person eating a diet high in protein and carbs—like the standard American diet (SAD)—you'll see "dirty" blood, full of yeast, bacteria, and mold—and blood cells actually transforming into those organisms. The irregular, poorly formed and damaged blood cells and red blood cells clump

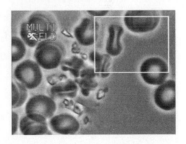

SAD diet live blood

together unnaturally. There are lots of white blood cells, trying to deal with all that mess. You'll see lots of crystals in the blood, which represent chelated acids. And you'll see formations of cellular debris, including crystallized acids as well as bacterias, yeasts, and molds and their wastes.

2. Healthy, alkaline live blood shows round, even, symmetrical individual blood cells in debris-free plasma. Notice the white blood

cells, which are active and streaming in the blood serum.

3. Dried blood from someone on the standard American diet has variations in color going from red to tan to brown to black. The white spots are protein masses from broken-down cells. You'll see fibrin monomer holding the blood together loosely, with breaks visible.

4. Healthy dried blood appears a consistent medium red throughout, and is held together tightly by black fibrin monomer. There is a solid mat of red blood cells.

The next set of illustrations comes from someone on a high-protein/ high-fat diet.

5. In the blood of someone on a high-protein, low-carb, high-fat diet you can see the red blood cells stacked together in "rouleau," which can cause higher than necessary blood pressure and poor circulation. There is also the black mass known technically as a fibrous thallus or colloid symplast. I refer to it as a "city of garbage," since it is an accumulation of bacteria, yeast, and sometimes even mold, and their associated acid waste products, all in a crystalline state. Its presence is also associated with circulation problems including cold hands and feet, muddled thinking, light-headedness, dizziness, and hypertension. As these masses build up in the blood they can cause heart attack or stroke. In addi-

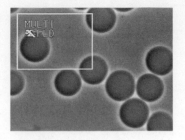

Healthy alkaline live blood

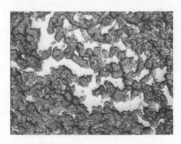

SAD dried blood

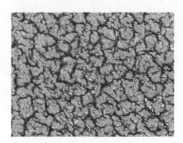

Healthy dried blood

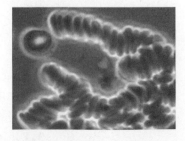

High-protein blood

tion, the blood of someone getting too much animal protein and not enough healthy fats will show lemon-shaped red blood cells, yellow or orange crystals of uric acid cells, and "shadow cells"— red blood cells with weak membranes due to lack of good fats in the diet.

6. This dried blood clot is typical of someone on a high animal protein diet. The black circle in the center of the blood drop is undigested proteins. The pasty white round protein masses indicate cellular breakdown.

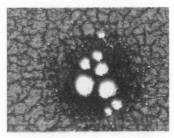

High-protein dried blood

The final set of illustrations are from someone who had been following a low-fat/high-carb diet.

7. I can always tell when I'm looking at the blood of someone on a low-fat diet because there are so many shadow cells, which can cause fatigue and anemia, and often come along with hormonal imbalances and poor immune function. Usually the person will be craving more protein and carbs. I'll also see fermenting red blood cells with white spots and blood cells

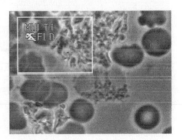

Live blood on low-fat/ high-carb

clumped together. There will be white and green crystals of acetylaldehyde, ethanol alcohol, and lactic acid. There will be lots of acid crystals that are clear and look like broken glass from the fermentation of the excess sugars. The crystals you see here are chelated with the alkalizing minerals like potassium, magnesium, and calcium, and even fats, in an effort to protect the cells against acid. These crystals can impair circulation, leading to hypertension, heart attack, or stroke. You'll also see red blood cells shaped like berries in blood that's not had enough fat and too many carbs, the result of weak cellular membranes caused by lack of good polyunsaturated fatty acids (omega-3s) or poor digestion of fats. Upon being digested, carbs leave behind tar, resin, and glue-like acid substances that cause adhesions—acid crystals—to impinge on blood vessels and lymphatic spaces as well as the intestinal villus, making everything sticky.

White blood cells are paralyzed by the high sugar content in the diet, or the inability to process sugar in the body—literally; they stay still when they should be streaming around, collecting garbage and keeping the internal environment clean.

8. The dried blood of someone on a low-fat/high-carb diet won't coagulate properly, leaving pasty white masses looking like jigsaw puzzles, or misty clouds. There are white protein masses (polymerizations) from cells that are broken down due to excess acidity, indicating too much sugar and too little good fats. They let you know cells are breaking down faster than they are being built up.

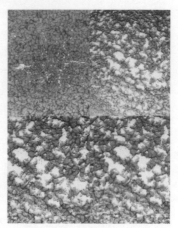

You'll also find a lack of fibrin monomer, a clotting protein that is the black that holds the conglomerate of red blood cells together.

Dried-blood on low-fat/ high-carb

Dark centers in the coagulated blood and circular white areas in the center of the coagulated blood—groups of proteins—indicate cellular breakdown.

WHAT'S IN YOUR BLOOD?

There's nothing like seeing the state of your own blood to get you going in an alkaline direction, and I encourage you to look into live blood analysis and dried blood testing with a certified microscopist in your area. (See Resources for a website to point you in the right direction.) Once you've cleaned up your blood, if you still need convincing (which I doubt actually; you'll probably be feeling too good to still be unsure) you could trying looking at your blood, live, half an hour to an hour after an acidic meal—pick one from any of the diet types listed earlier. You'd get dramatic results even after eating a single egg! You'd see in a most compelling fashion exactly what I'm talking about: the profound changes in your body, at the cellular level, depending on what you eat.

On the off chance you don't want to be your own guinea pig, I'll leave you with this pair of "before" and "after" pictures showing the effect of one meal of bacon and eggs.

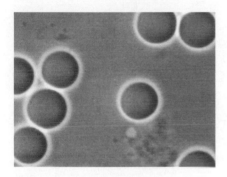 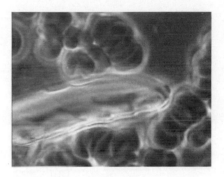

Before bacon and eggs   After bacon and eggs

Chapter 5

You Are What You Drink

Water is not only a mirror reflecting our mind—
water is the source of life.
—Masaru Emoto

The human body is 70 percent water. You've got roughly 10 to 13 gallons of water in your body. Water makes up 75 percent by volume of your muscles and heart, 83 percent of your brain and kidneys, 86 percent of your lungs, and 95 percent of your eyes. Even 22 percent of your bones are actually water. Most telling of all, your blood is 90 percent water. You are, quite literally, what you drink. If you don't drink enough—and most Americans don't—or if you drink the wrong things, you will compromise your body and your health. Your weight will be one obvious sign of that compromise. That's why I firmly believe the single most important thing you can do to not only be healthy but also to find and stay at your ideal weight is to drink good water—and plenty of it.

It turns out that isn't always as easy as it sounds, given the current state of our water supply. This chapter explains why most water isn't up to the job of keeping you healthy, then shows you how to make sure your water is. You'll also learn how to figure out how much water your body needs daily. I'll also explain a revolutionary water-purification and -processing technique that produces water that is ideal for the human body—water that will allow you to lose up to 1 pound *every day*.

THE DANGERS OF DEHYDRATION

Chances are you are among the 75 percent of Americans who are chronically dehydrated, meaning they don't get the eight, 8-ounce servings of water each day—about 2 liters—recommended by mainstream health experts. The average person gets only about *1* liter of fluid a day—much of it from acidic coffee, tea, and soft drinks, many of which actually *rob* the body of water. And to get even to that minimal level requires estimating the amount they get from food. Oh, and sometimes they get it from drinking actual water, though it is likely to be inadequate in quality as well as quantity. Fully 10 percent of respondents to a survey done for the Nutrition Information Center at Cornell Medical Center reported drinking no water at all!

For ideal health and weight, you need much more water—good water—as I'll detail later. The average adult loses about 2½ to 3 liters of fluid a day through sweating, breathing, urinating, moving, even sleeping, and the body becomes dehydrated if it isn't replaced.

If you don't get enough water, then you'll get fat. Simple as that. For one thing, even mild dehydration slows metabolism by as much as 3 percent. For another, we are so poorly attuned to our bodies' thirst signals that we interpret them as hunger pangs. That is, if we don't drink enough, we eat too much. Finally, if we don't get enough water, our bodies will actually retain water, and we'll feel bloated and uncomfortable—and look even fatter than strictly necessary! An acidic body pulls water into the tissues to try to neutralize the acids there.

Most important, the body uses water to neutralize acids, to dilute excess acid, and to literally wash them (and all toxins) out of the body via urine and sweat and through the bowels. Without enough water your body becomes too acidic and goes into preservation—fat-storing—mode. A drop of just over 2 percent in body water content is enough to make that happen. In case you think that sounds like such a big change that it is unlikely to ever happen to you, take note: It's not unusual to lose 2 percent of your body water during an average hour of exercise.

If that's not enough to get you to drink up, let me add that in addition to fat, not getting enough water will also make you sick and tired. In fact, lack of water is the number one cause of daytime fatigue. Without enough water, you won't have enough energy. You'll feel tired and weak.

That 2 percent drop in body water can result in a measurable decrease in physical performance. The acid that builds up in your tissues when you don't get enough water acts like a meat tenderizer, making your muscles flabby—and weak. Studies show that a 3 percent drop in water causes a 10 percent drop in muscle strength and an 8 percent drop in speed, as well as lower muscular endurance.

By the time you get to a 4 percent drop in body water, you'll experience dizziness—and a fall of as much as 30 percent in your capacity for physical labor. Drop another percentage point and you'll have problems with concentration, drowsiness, impatience, and headaches (one of the most common signs of dehydration, along with dry skin). Losing another percent can cause your heart to race and your body's temperature regulation to go out of whack. Hit 7 percent, and you could collapse.

Even in the earliest stages, dehydration can also lead to muddled thinking, short-term memory problems, trouble with basic math and expressing yourself verbally, and difficulty focusing on a computer screen or printed page. Light-headedness and cold hands and feet can also result. The list goes on: anxiety, irritability, depression, sugar cravings, and cramps.

As for making you sick: When the dehydration gets a little more severe, symptoms include acid reflux (heartburn), joint and back pain, migraines, fibromyalgia, constipation, colitis, and angina. Serious dehydration is linked with asthma, allergies, diabetes, hypertension, and such skin problems as eczema, rashes, spots, blemishes, and acne. Degenerative conditions including morbid obesity, heart disease, and cancer are all linked with serious long-term dehydration. If you lose 15 to 20 percent of your body's water, it can be immediately life-threatening.

In short: Lack of water can kill you.

In fact, although you could go about thirty days without eating, you can't live seventy-two hours without water. Your body uses as much water in cold weather as it does in warm, and as much when you are sleeping as when you are awake. In an average day, even with physical activity or environmental extremes (like a hot and/or dry climate), and with no particular drains on your body's water supply (like air travel, or time in a high-rise building), you can lose 1 percent of the water in your body. Although the most serious symptoms listed here don't come from spending an hour or a day with low levels of water in your tank, most people exist in a chronic state of low-level dehydration for most of their lives. No wonder so very many of us are fat and sick and tired!

HYDRATE FOR HEALTH

Fortunately, this is a relatively easy problem to solve. Finding the right water may take some doing, as you'll see, but essentially you just need to drink up! Those who do provide their bodies with this crucial element for normal performance, in everything from temperature regulation and toxin excretion to joint lubrication and fat metabolism. Water helps process just about every biological, mechanical, and chemical action that takes place in your body. It cushions and protects vital organs, transports nutrients within each cell, and dispels acidic wastes. Your lungs need water to humidify the air they move. The digestive system uses several gallons of water daily to process food. Your brain needs water to perform the chemical reactions required to run your body. Your pancreas uses water to alkalize food coming out of the stomach and into the intestines. Water keeps your skin soft and supple, increases oxygen in the blood, and maintains normal electrical properties of the cells, improving cell-to-cell communication.

One study published in the *Journal of the American Dietetic Association* showed that women who drank more than five glasses of water a day had 45 percent less risk of colon cancer. Another study from the same journal showed a 50 percent decrease in the risk of bladder cancer in people who drank 2.5 quarts of water daily and a

79 percent drop in the risk of breast cancer. A survey of over three thousand American adults conducted at The New York Hospital—Cornell Medical Center indicates that eight to ten glasses of water a day could significantly reduce back and joint pain for up to 80 percent of sufferers. Drinking plenty of water also helps prevent kidney stones.

Perhaps of most immediate interest to you as you work on losing weight: A University of Washington study showed that one glass of water shut down hunger pangs for nearly all dieters in the study. And German researchers found that drinking water increases the rate at which you burn calories. Just 2 cups of water increased metabolic rate by almost a third—and it stayed up for about half an hour. When they reported their findings in the *Journal of Clinical Endocrinology and Metabolism,* they calculated that getting an additional 1.5 liters of water a day for a year would mean burning off an extra 17,400 calories—or about 5 pounds.

THE RIGHT WATER

For all the wonders of water, the *wrong kind* of water can actually make you sick, tired—and fat. Your water, like just about everything else you take in, must be electron-rich and alkaline. Sadly, almost all

---

David

I'm forty-eight years old, originally from Iowa, and live in England now. I lost 20 pounds, going from 180 to 160, in one month just by drinking water with pH drops (3 liters a day), cutting out meat and dairy, and eating more salads. I am still in a transition stage; having eaten meat for more than four decades, it does take some time to adjust! I have a ways to go yet to be vegetarian, but with Shelley Young's recipes it should be an easy transition.

of the readily available water is acidic, and this will make your body acidic and send it into the whole fat-holding cycle of self-preservation. And that's while your body *should* be able to use the water you supply it with to neutralize and wash away acids! With acidic water, you're never going to reach your ideal weight or your ideal state of health. But when you properly hydrate your body with electron-rich alkaline water, you are providing what your body needs to keep its cells healthy and pH balanced—without having to pull neutralizing agents from elsewhere in the body, where they have other jobs to do. Body cells are only as healthy as the fluids they are bathed in.

Okay, you're ready for a drink, and you've got a glass of tap water, or a bottle of water from the store. It looks clear and good. It may even taste good. But is it really good for you? Is it even safe to drink? Is it acidic or alkaline? Is it going to speed you to your ideal weight, or keep you stuck in entirely the wrong zone of the scale? Just by looking and tasting, you have no real way to know. What I've uncovered by testing waters from around the country and around the globe, however, is that your odds are low of having in front of you right now something you *really* want to drink. The most important characteristics of truly healthy water are its purity, pH, electron activity, and molecular structure. I'll explain a bit about each below.

Purity

First of all, you must be sure your water is pure and safe to drink. And just because it came out of your tap, or out of a store-bought bottle, or from a public water supply doesn't make it so. Physicians for Social Responsibility reports that over 75,000 toxic synthetic and chemical compounds can be identified in this country's water sources, though only a fraction of them are targeted for regulation. Indeed, the Environmental Protection Agency (EPA) recently documented approximately 83,000 violations of water quality standards by municipal water systems, featuring over 21,000 contaminants—organic and inorganic—over the past thirty years, almost 200 of them already proven to be linked with adverse health effects. Industry and agriculture cause a lot of this contamination, but much of it can be traced back to everyday products like lawn chemicals, prescription drugs, gasoline, and household cleaners.

More than 240 million Americans use water from contaminated public water systems every day, according to the Natural Resources Defense Council (NRDC). The Centers for Disease Control and Prevention (CDC) estimates that almost 1 million people in America fall ill annually from water contaminated with harmful microorganisms—and about 900 die.

Turning to bottled water won't necessarily help. Among other things, many bottled waters are simply bottled tap water. (See the chart on page 65 for more details about the characteristics of the many bottled waters I've tested.)

The truth is, there doesn't seem to be any naturally good water left on the planet. Once glacial melt must have been just about ideal, or rainwater, or spring water near the source, or high mountain streams. But in today's industrial age of acid rain, air pollution, contaminated groundwater, and ocean garbage dumping, you can't get the water your body really needs without some modification.

A high-quality filter is definitely in order to make sure your water is free of such various impurities as undesirable chemicals, trace elements, and microorganisms. I think a distiller or an electronic water purifier would be your best bet. (Or buy distilled water, available at any grocery store.) Setting up the equipment to purify your water at home will run you about $400 to $1,500. I recommend the ReGenesis purifier, which filters and ionizes water, or the Living Water Machine distiller by Crystal Clear (see Resources).

pH

To be truly healthful, your water must also be alkaline. Pure distilled water ranks an even 7 on the pH scale. Anything above 7 is alkaline, and so better than acidic water, but to get the full benefits of alkaline water—neutralizing the acids that make you fat—I recommend water that's at least 9.5 on the pH scale (and as high as 11.5 to 12.5 in cases of serious health conditions, including extreme obesity). Most water today is more acidic than neutral. Imagine: You're drink-

FILTERS TO FORGET ABOUT

In looking for a water filter you'll find a vast array of technologies available. Several of the most common, however, can't provide you with the water your body really needs, so you should pass them over in favor of the better options described earlier:

- A simple charcoal filter for tap water may improve the taste and does remove some unwanted elements, but it can't eliminate all the stuff you need to be concerned about.
- Deionizers don't remove synthetic chemicals, and the resin beds used to filter the water are notorious breeding grounds for microorganisms.
- Chlorination doesn't remove any chemicals. In fact, it adds a potentially health-damaging one!
- Ultraviolet (UV) machines don't target all worrisome microorganisms and are high maintenance besides.
- Ozonation release protons and acids (bad) along with the ozone (good), and the systems are inefficient and expensive.

ing acidic water, requiring your body to draw down its stores of alkaline substances even more just to neutralize water that by rights *should* be neutral in the first place—when you *could* be saving those stores by providing good alkaline water. And don't be fooled by "pH-balanced" claims like the ones on certain bottled water labels: "Naturally pH balanced at 7.2." True, that is just the slightest bit alkaline, and it is certainly better than acidic water. But to really reap the benefits of alkaline water, that pH just isn't high enough.

Drinking alkaline water washes away acids and wastes, helping your whole body stay alkaline. By providing alkaline water to neutralize and remove acid from the tissues, you'll stop the body from gleaning alkaline substances from other body parts to do the job—like leeching calcium from your bones. Acidic water could contain toxic metal ions, like lead, cadmium, and mercury, which in excess can cause serious health issues. Conversely, alkaline water may be filled with alkaline minerals your body needs, like calcium, magnesium, and potassium, and in the only form your body can absorb (ionic). And negative microforms won't be able to thrive in an environment supplied with plenty of alkaline water.

Fortunately, there's an easy way to make sure your water is alkaline: To each liter of water (preferably ionized or distilled), add 16 drops of 2 percent sodium chlorite, or 2 to 3 teaspoons of sodium bicarbonate (plain old baking soda) or sodium silicate. Ask at your natural food store for sodium silicate or sodium chlorite. See chapter 9 for more details on pH drops.

Electron Activity/Energy/Energy Potential

To reach your ideal weight, your water must be energized. Energized water is saturated with electrons, highly charged, and full of potential energy. You already know that alkaline water has a negative charge because of all its electrons, whereas acids are dominated by positively charged protons, and that it is the attraction of electrons to the protons that neutralizes harmful acids. Here I'll explain the two ways to measure the electron activity, or energy potential, of water: ORP and rH2.

The value of ORP (oxidative reduction potential) quantifies the amount of energy in your water (or anything else) by numbering its electrons. It is expressed in millivolts (mV). Make sure your water registers in negative millivolts. To get you to your ideal weight, your water should have an ORP of at least −50 mV. (And you don't want to go beyond −1,250 mV, and as you get close to that you only want a small amount of it on any given day.) That means there will be sufficient electron activity to neutralize excess acids that would otherwise cause your body to gain or hold weight. Most tap water comes in at about +500 mV.

Consider rH2 (reduction of hydrogen; sometimes called "redox") as sort of a backup measure to ORP. rH2 is measured on a scale, just the way pH is. The rH2 scale ranges from 0 to 44, with 22 being

Andy

I was going through life overweight—and just not caring anymore. I'd tried so many programs and nothing ever worked. Until I heard about this plan. In just five months 60 pounds came right off, and I have stayed at my ideal weight of 160 for over

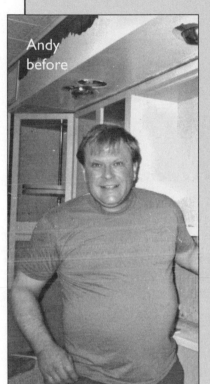

Andy before

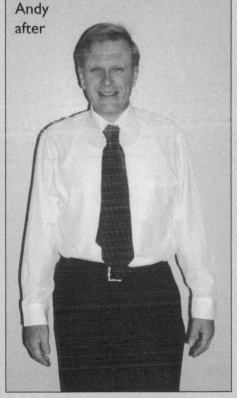

Andy after

two years now. My cholesterol has dropped 100 points, my blood pressure is normal, and I take no medications. I love this way of life and have amazed my friends—and doctor—with how young and good looking I am now!

neutral; the lower the number, the greater the concentration of electrons. With each step, the number of electrons increases by a factor of 10; water with rH2 of 22 has 10 times more electrons than water at 23. An increase of just two places on the scale, then, means 100 times fewer electrons. You want your water to have an rH2 of 22 or less. Unfortunately, most municipalities have, on average, an rH2 of 30 or greater. That's 100 million fewer electrons than you're aiming for. Our water is not providing us with the energy we need to be healthy and maintain a healthy weight.

You already know the solution to this dilemma, however. Adding the sodium chlorite, bicarbonate, or silicate to your water as described earlier increases not only pH but also electron activity. These substances react with and release oxygen in the water, increasing its energy potential.

Molecular Structure

The final critical characteristic of water to consider is molecular structure. In most tap and bottled water, H_2O molecules tend to cluster together in groups of 10 to 20. Electron activity occurs on the surface of a molecule, and as molecules cluster together, the total surface area decreases, thereby decreasing electron activity. Conversely, the smaller the clusters formed, the higher the electron activity. Furthermore, large clusters of molecules can't permeate cell membranes very well, and so can't hydrate the cells from the inside. The smaller the size of the cluster of molecules, the better able the water is to hydrate the cell and the more oxygen it can provide.

Your water should have no more than 5 to 6 molecules clustered together. Ideally you'd get monomolecular water—each molecule stands as an individual, without clustering. Two cutting-edge processing methods can provide you with properly structured water.

PAW, or plasma-activated water, uses electromagnetic fields and ultrasound and UV radiation to break down the molecular clusters and increase the electrical potential of ordinary tap water without chemicals or heat, creating highly electrically charged water with smaller molecule clusters of 1 to 2 molecules (vs. 10 to 24 in most tap or well water). Most tap water emerges from the machine with a pH of 9.5, an ORP of –250 mV and an rH2 of 19.5. The increase in electron activity remains stable for several weeks—you don't have to drink this water immediately upon making it to receive its benefits the way you do with plain ionized water. And testing by the National Testing Laboratories in Cleveland, Ohio, has found PAW to exceed every standard for levels of bacteria, metals, non-metallic inorganic chemicals, organic chemicals, pesticides, herbicides, and polychlorinated biphenyls (PCBs).

PAM, or plasma-activated micro-ionized water, I make with a machine of my own invention, on which I have a patent pending. (Check the pH Miracle website—see Resources—for up-to-date availability.) Essentially, PAM takes PAW one step further, adding a micro-ionization process that increases the amount of electrons in the water. It creates fully monomolecular water, the only process to

GOOD WATER

Water that will help you live at your ideal weight, and in general good health, has

- no impurities (pesticides or other chemicals, metals like arsenic or lead or other toxins, organisms or contaminants including bacteria, yeast, mold, and algae).
- a pH of at least 9.5.
- an ORP of –50 mV or better.
- an rH2 of 22 or less.
- a maximum of 5 or 6 molecules per cluster.

Water like this isn't just going to come out of your tap, and you can't just buy a bottle of it. But by investing in a PAM or PAW machine, or distilling or ionizing your water, or buying distilled water, then adding pH drops as detailed in chapter 9, you can provide your body with what it is truly thirsty for.

do so; thus, no other water can provide as much energy potential or be as easily absorbed by the body and the cells. PAM has a pH between 9.5 and 12.5, an ORP between −50 and −1,250 mV, and is stable for several months.

Alternately, the adding of the sodium drops or powders already described can help reduce the size of the molecular clusters.

WATER, WATER EVERYWHERE, AND NOT A DROP TO DRINK

The statistics earlier in the chapter should be enough to make you suspicious of the healthfulness of your tap water. But turning to bottled water isn't any guarantee of getting really good water. In North America, more than 70 percent of people drink bottled water, downing over 13 billion liters each year. (Though we are still relative slouches in this area, compared with the 90 percent of French and Italian people who drink bottled water.) You have more than seven hundred brands from around the world to choose from. But whether you choose spring water, artesian water, mineral water, sparkling water, well water, or municipal drinking water (which is what you're getting in most of those bottled waters anyway), you are most likely getting proton-saturated, acidic water. Water with no energy. Water that will actually *steal* energy away from your body, rather than contributing to good health.

Approximately 80 percent of bottled water brands are processed waters—municipal or tap water that has been run through a filtration system for impurities and chemicals. Both Aquafina (from Pepsi) and Dasani (from Coke), for example, are simply bottled from municipal water supplies. More than half of bottled waters around the world are exempt from governmental standards; they don't have to live up to even the minimal standards tap water is regulated by. Buying bottled water is no assurance that it is any safer or healthier than tap water. And in some cases, your own tap water would be a better choice. Ask any company you buy water from for a complete lab analysis of their water to see if it is good for you. The companies won't be able to tell you about all the characteristics explained in this chapter, but it will be good for them to know people are asking—and they can at least tell you the measurements (in ppm, parts per million) of certain chemicals and metals in the water.

I tested more than sixty of the most popular and (supposedly!) best bottled waters from around the world to see if any met my criteria for pH and electron activity. The results listed in the following chart should be more than enough to make you very interested in the next section, on ways to filter, charge, and structure your water yourself: the only two that had a pH above 9.5 carried a positive charge. In fact, I found only *one* with a negative charge! And of course you will be expected to pay top dollar for all of them. But all water is most definitely not created equal. You need to make sure you are drinking high pH water with extra electrons for increased energy.

Brand or Type	Source and Features	pH	ORP (mV)	rH2
Propel Fitness Water	Processed water with minerals added	3.37	+305	27.05
San Pellegrino	San Pellegrino, Italy spring water^e	4.49	+449	28.49
llanllyr Source	West Wales, UK spring water^e drawn from beneath the organic fields of llanllyr	4.75	+447	28.47
Perrier	Perrier, France	4.91	+478	28.78
Pellegrino	San Pellegrino, Italy sparkling natural mineral water	5.28	+392	27.92
Hawaiian Islands	Natural filtered spring water	5.36	+618	30.18
Aqua Diva	Tuscany, Italy natural mineral water from an artesian well^a	5.78	+611	30.11
New York City municipal water	Filtered tap water	5.81	+440	28.40
Aquafina	Filtered municipal water	5.96	+431	28.31
Badoit	St. Galmier, France natural sparkling water from a deep water table through a 1,500-foot fissure	6.0	+426	28.26
Ferrarelle	Mountains of southern Italy natural spring water	6.1	+428	28.28
Valverde	Italian Alps spring water^e	6.22	+402	28.02

Brand or Type	Source and Features	pH	ORP (mV)	rH2
Spa	Reine River, France spring water[e]	6.23	+418	28.18
Deja Blue	North American purified or filtered tap water	6.28	+434	28.34
Deer Park	Allegheny Mountains near Deer Park, Maryland spring water	6.31	+644	30.41
Poland Spring	Spring water[d]	6.31	+390	26.90
Hawaii Water	Reverse osmosis–filtered spring water[e]	6.38	+386	27.86
Chatledon	Auvergne, France A natural spring mineral water, one of the first bottled waters; presented in 1654 to Louis XIV to help cure his gout	6.58	+358	27.58
Fiji	Fiji Islands spring water[e]	6.65	+ 406	28.06
Blue Moon	Processed filtered tap water	6.65	+365	27.65
Voss	Norway artesian[a] water	6.67	+357	27.57
Penta	Micro-ionized[c]	6.7	+789	31.89
Fonyodi	Budapest, Hungary natural spring water	6.80	+502	29.02
Arrowhead	Spring water[e]	6.83	+359	27.59
Eon	Natural springs, Mount Shasta deep ice pack water, reverse osmosis and carbon filtered, ozonated,[b] no heat or added minerals or chemical stabilizers	6.84	+578	29.78
Laurisia	Italy melted snow that seeps up through a volcanic rock grotto	6.87	+398	27.98
Calistoga	Mayacmas, Sierra, Nevada, and Polomar mountains near San Diego, California spring water[e]	6.93	+404	28.04
Crystal Geyser	California's Mount Whitney spring water	6.93	+404	28.04
Lissa	Italy natural mineral water[d]	6.96	+398	27.98
Smart Water	Vapor-distilled[f] water with minerals added	6.97	+368	27.68

Brand or Type	Source and Features	pH	ORP (mV)	rH2
Volvic	Natural mineral water[d] filtered through volcanic rock	7.07	+407	28.07
Whistler Water	Ozonated[b] glacier water	7.18	+419	28.19
Dasani	North America purified tap water	7.2	+378	27.78
Nariwa	Japan spring water from Magnetic Mountain	7.30	+303	27.03
Tynant	Bethania, Wales, UK natural mineral water[d]	7.30	+396	27.96
Scottish Natural Mineral Water	Campsie Falls, Lennoxtown, Scotland natural mineral water[d]	7.36	+408	28.08
Ice Age	Ozonated[b] glacier water	7.39	+378	27.78
Thames River	London Thames River	7.42	+405	28.05
Buxton	Buxton, England artesian water drawn from 4,500 feet underground	7.42	+400	28
Brecon Carreg	Brecon National Park, Nottingham, England spring water[e]	7.42	+391	27.91
Absopure	Irish Hills, Michigan spring water, ozonated, ultraviolet	7.48	+455	28.75
Evian	Evian, France	7.53	+390	27.90
Natural Value	Sacramento, California spring water[e]	7.54	+381	27.81
Zephyrhills	Spring water	7.57	+362	27.62
Cloud Juice	"800 drops of Tasmanian rainwater"	7.58	+367	27.67
Treewater	Pickens, West Virginia reverse osmosis or filtered water and ozonated water	7.65	+453	28.53
Barraute municipal water	Quebec, Canada first place in municipal waters at the 2002 International Water Tasting Awards	7.79	+483	28.83
Dannon	Natural spring water	7.84	+546	29.46
Waiwera	New Zealand artesian[a]	7.87	+356	27.56
Canadian Mountain	Melted glacier	7.96	+364	27.64

Brand or Type	Source and Features	pH	ORP (mV)	rH2
Aqua Hydrate	Utah purified water with minerals added	7.96	+358	27.58
Vittel	Vosges, France spring water[e]	7.98	+402	27.98
Coumayeur	Mont Blanc Massif (in the Alps) natural mineral water[d]	8.02	+410	28.10
Palm Springs municipal water	Filtered and chlorinated tap water	8.13	+515	29.15
Acqua Panna	Tuscan Apennines of Northern Italy, 25 miles north of Florence natural spring water	8.20	+523	29.23
Iceberg Water	Newfoundland melted icebergs	8.31	+326	27.36
Essentia Water	Micro-Ionized[b]	8.57	+ 58	22.58
Evermore	Artesian[a]	9.23	−57	21.43
pH Miracle Water I	Plasma activated micro-ionized	9.5	−250	19.50
Trinity Geothermal Water Original	Artesian[a]	9.55	+330	27.30
Regenesis Water	Micro-ionized	9.8	−78	21.22
Trinity Natural Mineral Supplement	Artesian[a]	9.88	+316	27.16
pH Miracle Water II	Plasma-activated micro-ionized	11.5	−750	14.50
pH Miracle Water III	Plasma-activated micro-ionized	12.5	−1,250	8.50

[a] Water from an artesian well—a well that taps a water-bearing underground layer of rock or sand, in which the water level stands above the top of the aquifer (porous rock that acts as a natural filter to keep out microforms and other toxins).
[b] Ozonated water contains a particular form of oxygen, which breaks down into another form that fights bacteria and other microbes, including yeast.
[c] Micro-ionized: see passages on PAM and PAW, previously.
[d] Mineral water must contain at least 250 parts per million of dissolved minerals and trace elements thought to be healthful. No minerals can be added; the minerals in the bottled version must match the water at the source. Note that calcium, magnesium, and potassium are all alkaline, but that iron, manganese, copper, and zinc are all acidic; so you need to be very careful about the amounts you get of them, and the form they come in.
[e] Spring water comes from an underground formation through which the water flows naturally to the earth's surface, and can be collected only at the spring or through a hole bored into an underground spring.
[f] See Purity section, page 57.

DRINKING WATER

Water sold for human consumption must contain no added sweeteners or chemical additives other than flavors, extracts, or essences that comprise less than 1 percent of the product's final weight. (Otherwise, it is no longer considered water, but a soft drink.) Drinking water must be sugar-free and either salt-free or very low in sodium.

HOW MUCH WATER DO WE NEED?

If, like most people, you drink only when you feel thirsty, you're not getting enough water. Your body loses 2 to 3 liters of water daily through normal activity (breathing, sleeping, walking around), and you need to be sure not only to replace that but also to further hydrate your body. Thirst lags far behind your body's need for water and is an inadequate signal of your body's full spectrum of needs. In fact, what thirst indicates is a mild state of dehydration. If you rely solely on thirst to replenish your water when you exercise, it takes up to twenty-four hours for your body to return to proper hydration status.

As a rule of thumb, you need to get 1 liter of electron rich, alkaline water every day per each 40 pounds of body weight—per 30 pounds for those engaging in moderate exercise like the program in this book. For someone weighing 160 pounds, that's 4 to 5 liters a day—a gallon or more. For someone 210 pounds, up to 7 liters a day is required. As part of your routine, you should drink 8 ounces of water before you work out, 4 ounces every 15 minutes or so while you exercise, and 8 ounces again about half an hour after you finish exercising. You should also weigh yourself before and after exercise to make sure you've replaced all lost fluids. It's not unusual to lose up to 2 percent of your body water during an hour of exercise (as much as a pound!).

A person who drinks only 2 liters a day will not get the results that a person who drinks 5 liters a day could expect. A person who also makes adjustments to what he or she eats according to the guidelines in this book will do better and faster than someone who only drinks water but still eats acidic foods. In large part, your results are up to you!

HOW MUCH DO *I* NEED?

Take a minute right now to figure out how much water you actually drink each day. Don't count soda, coffee, milk, juice, tea, and any other flavored, carbonated, sweetened, alcoholic, or caffeinated liquids, all of which are acidic and proton saturated—just water! How many 8-ounce cups? How many liters? (There being roughly 4 cups to the liter.)

Now, based on your current weight, how much water should you drink each day?

Finally, how are you going to get from here to there? Start out slowly, and gradually build up to your goal. Make a plan for yourself about how much more water you are going to drink each day, until you build up to your target. Say you're drinking 2 liters a day right now (which would already put you ahead of most Americans, in line with general medical recommendations), but since you weigh 210 pounds you should really be drinking more like 7. Decide to add half a liter to your intake each day and in ten days you'll be on target. Tomorrow you'll drink 2 liters and 2 cups, the day after that 3 liters, and so on. Or, up your water by a liter a day to get yourself there in just five days. You get the idea.

Write your plan down. Commit to it. Note your daily progress. Drink up!

DRINK MORE, WEIGH LESS

Doctors and nutritionists will say that losing weight by drinking water is not possible. And that is true—with the water that is currently out there! But with sufficient amounts of electron-rich, alkaline-structured water you make yourself, you can lose up to a pound a day.

(Even mainstream experts would agree that if we drank water instead of soft drinks we'd shave off pounds. The average American guzzles 44 gallons of soft drinks per year, about one 16-ounce bottle each and every day. That's easily enough to add a few pounds every year.)

Getting the right water in the right amount is the single most important part of the pH Miracle Living plan for healthy weight loss. Fully hydrating the body with good water is the quickest and easiest way to reach and maintain your ideal weight.

HOW TO DRINK YOUR WAY TO IDEAL WEIGHT

- Drink only "good" water (PAM or PAW or distilled or ionized with pH drops or sodium bicarbonate).
- Drink at least 1 liter of good water each day for every 30 pounds of body weight.
- Drink 1 liter of good water when you first get up in the morning. This helps to flush out your kidneys, bladder, and bowels as well as rehydrates and energizes or charges your body with extra electrons.
- Drink one 16-ounce glass every hour, or 1 liter every two hours.
- Drink most of your water between meals.
- Drink at habitual times throughout the day; don't wait until you feel thirsty or hungry.
- Drink an extra liter of water for each hour of exercise.
- Drink your water warm to ease congestion or constipation.
- Drink 16 ounces at the end of each day.

Chapter 6

Fat Is Your Friend

A truth's initial commotion is directly proportional to how deeply the lie was believed. It wasn't the world being round that agitated people, but that the world wasn't flat. When a well-packaged web of lies has been sold gradually to the masses over generations, the truth will seem utterly preposterous and its speaker a raving lunatic.
—Dresden James

In order to lose weight, you're going to need to increase the amount of quality fat in your diet. That's right: Eat more fat. I'm going to give you a moment to let that sink in. It may take a little while to undo the many years of preaching about "low-fat" diets we've all lived through over the past two decades or so. You've heard for years that the way to drop fat off your body is to cut fat out of your diet. I'm here to stand up for a radically different view.

The truth is, fat isn't, by definition, bad for you. Fat is, in fact, your friend. This chapter moves beyond the fact that fat storage deposits on your body are actually saving your life to examine the importance of including fat—the right fat—in your diet to ensure healthy, permanent weight loss. You'll receive a variety of benefits to your health—permanent weight loss prime among them. In fact, fats are the single most important food you can eat to regulate your weight!

Reading this chapter will let you see fats in a whole new light. To wit: Fats are the most important food you will eat to regulate your weight. And low- or no-fat diets will make you fat. Eating fat does *not* make you fat. Rather, it's eating *acid* that piles on the pounds. The solution to being overweight, then, is not to stop eating fats, but to stop eating acids—and start eating good fats! An array of beneficial fats should be an integral part of every one of your daily meals. This chapter shows you why and points you in the direction of how (more specifics of which you'll find in later chapters).

THE BENEFITS OF FAT

A healthy adult human body is 20 percent fat. It's a crucial—and very busy—20 percent. After oxygen and water, fat is the next most important component of a healthy, fit body. Fat, a critical component of cellular membranes, is necessary for building healthy cells. Fat is crucial in hormone production and joint lubrication. Fat provides protection from physical impact, including insulating and padding your organs. Fat helps keep blood moving smoothly through the circulatory system. Several crucial vitamins are fat soluble, meaning they are only available to the body if bound to fat. Your body simply cannot function properly without a good supply of fat.

Fat has two functions in the body that are particularly important for achieving and maintaining your ideal weight. First, as I mentioned previously: The body uses fat to buffer, or neutralize, acids. Your body needs fat to maintain the blood and extracellular fluids at an ideal pH of 7.365. Providing your body with the right amounts of the right fats will allow the fat to bind with any excess acids and eliminate them from the body. (Too much acid, though, and the fat gets stored instead.)

One way fat helps neutralize acid is actually by creating cholesterol. When acids build up in the body, it signals the liver to use fat to make cholesterol. The more acidic the body, the more cholesterol is made. Specifically, the liver (which is responsible for 80 percent of our cholesterol—what we get from our diets accounts for only 20 percent) makes LDL cholesterol, famous as "bad" cholesterol because it makes up the plaque inside your arteries that can eventually impede blood flow. The plaque is actually protective, however, saving your arteries from the ravages of acids. Without it, without the cholesterol, the acids could burn holes right through the arteries throughout your circulatory system, and you could bleed to death. Turns out cholesterol is your friend, too. Ultimately, the buildup of too much plaque does become dangerous in and of itself, fulfilling the promise of cholesterol's bad reputation: high risk of heart attack and stroke. The real problem, however, is not the cholesterol, but the acid! Eliminate the acid, and you don't have to worry about cholesterol or plaque. And there goes one of the biggest arguments (cholesterol control) in favor of low-fat diets!

The second key point regarding eating fat and losing weight is using fat as fuel. Most human bodies burn sugar (carbohydrates) for fuel. Basically, that's what is readily at hand. Given the chance, though, the body will run on fat, which is a much cleaner, more efficient fuel. One of the aims of the pH Miracle Living plan is to teach your body to use fat as fuel. Fat creates six times more energy than burning sugar, or protein, while using much less energy in the process. Furthermore, burning fat results in much lower levels of acid waste products. Metabolism is one of the major sources of acid in the body, so slashing the amount of acids produced in this way goes a long way toward balancing your body's pH—and its weight.

WHY LOW-FAT HASN'T WORKED— AND HOW IT HAS HURT

For decades we've been advised to slash the fat from our diets. It seemed to make sense. Eating fat makes you fat, the argument went. If you don't want to be fat, don't eat fat. There's just one problem: It hasn't worked. Well, two, really: It isn't true.

Since we as a nation embarked on a quest to get rid of fat in our diets and so off our bodies, we've gotten even fatter, and at an alarmingly steep rate of increase to boot. For one thing, we didn't successfully reduce our fat intake at all—from 1980 to 1991 it remained pretty much the same as it began, at about 81 grams a day per person. But we compensated for the fat we cut out (*thought* we cut out) by increasing the amount of carbohydrates and animal proteins we ate. What we did manage to do was cut the percentage of calories from fat slightly—but only because we increased the number of calories we ate each day! And the sugary foods we loaded up on are all acidic.

Even people who really do decrease their fat intake can't expect to lose weight. In a six-week study at the Mayo Clinic, overweight women followed a diet with 45 percent of its calories from fat for two weeks, then switched to a low-fat diet with the same number of calories (mainly from additional carbohydrates) for a month. Not a single participant lost weight or body fat. Researchers could also detect no change in metabolic rate. According to the Mayo team: "NO effect of the four-week, low-fat diet could be detected."

Furthermore, insufficient fat in your diet can cause a variety of health problems. Your skin may suffer, for one thing, as acids are eliminated through "the third kidney" rather than being bound to fats and eliminated through the bowels or urinary system. As acids escape through the skin, you may have blotchy, dry skin, rashes, and cracks at the corners of the mouth. Without enough fat, you'll have brittle hair and weak nails. More important, your neurotransmitters can't function correctly without sufficient essential fatty acids, potentially interfering with your nerve function. Diets too low in fat have been linked to depression and mood disorders, and heart disease. Without the fats essential to cell membranes, you'll have weak body and blood cells, and associated problems including anemia, poor circulation, inappropriate clotting, and high blood pressure. Without healthy cell membranes, your body is at extreme risk of cellular breakdown leading to serious illness or disease. In short, fat is essential, and to limit or eliminate it sets the stage for serious degenerative consequences.

THE FAILURES OF FAT

By now you may be wondering why I'm bothering to tout the benefits of fat when everyone knows Americans are already experts on getting plenty of fat in their diets. And on the surface, that's true: Americans currently get about 30 percent of their calories from fat—a drop from 40 percent in 1955, and in line with official nutritional recommendations. But these are largely the wrong kinds of fats—hydrogenated and trans fats. Still, this plan's recommendation of 40 percent of calories from fat will look shocking to many people who have been exposed to low- or no-fat fad diets for so long.

A vast body of mainstream studies have correlated high-fat diets with increased risk of heart disease, stroke, diabetes, cancer, and, of course, overweight and obesity. When we look at the fatty typical American diet, it is easy to see how it was concluded that fat is bad for you.

But that's missing the real problem. What's bad for you is not the fat per se—it's the typical American diet! (Nutrition professionals refer to it as the standard American diet, or SAD, for short. Sad indeed!) The vast majority of the fat most people get in this country comes from acidic, artery-clogging hydrogenated saturated and trans fats. The picture changes dramatically when the fats in question come from the healthful options available. And trying to lose weight by eating more fat, like trying to lose weight by eating less fat, will be doomed to failure unless you also reduce or eliminate the acidic foods and drinks that are the true culprits.

THE FOUR FATS

The key to eating fat to lose weight is understanding the different types of fats: saturated, trans, monounsaturated, and polyunsaturated. Any given fat or oil has a mixture of these types of fat, and are classified according to which type is predominant. As you'll see, there are big differences in the effects these fats have on your body. But at baseline, all these fats are much the same. A fat molecule contains carbon atoms bonded to other carbon atoms; the number of carbons in the chain varies by the specific fat. Fats are grouped into types depending on how many of those carbon atoms bond with a pair of hydrogen atoms. If every carbon attaches to two hydrogens, the result is a saturated fat (i.e., it is saturated with hydrogen). If all but one carbon bonds to a hydrogen pair, it forms a monounsaturated fat; more than one pair of hydrogens missing results in a polyunsaturated fat. Trans fats are basically artificially super-saturated fats unusable by the body. As you'll recall, the more saturated with hydrogen a substance is, the higher its positive charge, and the more acidic it is. In your quest for an alkaline—and ideal weight—body, you need to take in negatively charged foods, including fats. Furthermore, the more saturated a fat is to begin with, the less able it is to bind with acids, and to get them out of circulation in your body—there's just less room on the bus. Saturated fats are not much use as acid buffers, though the body can use naturally occurring forms for energy.

Saturated Fat

Most fats from animal sources—dairy, meat, poultry, eggs—are saturated. A few vegetable fats, notably coconut, palm, and safflower oils, are also rich in saturated fats. One hallmark of saturated fats is that they are solid at room temperature. Saturated fats can fuel your body, but they can't buffer acids.

Most Americans get plenty of saturated fats from the animal products they eat. Besides that, the body can make its own saturated fats. Your body needs some saturated fats to make necessary cholesterol. The fat layer under your skin, providing insulation, is almost entirely made of saturated fats. But so are the plaques that form inside blood vessels that can eventually block the flow of blood.

In the 1950s, researchers established saturated fat's bad reputation, and to this day it is generally equated with weight gain, clogged arteries, high blood pressure, high cholesterol, heart disease, and stroke. But it isn't really saturated fats that are bad for you—it's what happens to those fats during processing, cooking, and metabolism. In fact, some saturated fats actually help prevent those conditions and are essential to good health.

There are twelve kinds of saturated fats, most of them known as long-chain fatty acids because of their long (about 20 atoms) carbon chains. Saturated fats in meat are long-chain, and they don't break down easily unless heated, so the body can't make good use of them as fuel. And when long-chain saturated fats are heated enough to break down, either during processing or cooking, trans fats are formed (the dangers of which are explained next).

Far better are saturated fats from plant sources. Saturated fat from coconut and palm oils are medium-chain or sometimes short-chain fats, and they break down at body temperature so they can be used for energy. (The saturated fats in coconut—lauric oils—are very similar to what appears in human breast milk, the most perfect food on the planet!) You must be sure to get cold-pressed coconut oil, however, as processing it with heat creates trans fats (see below). Theoretically the same would be true for palm oil, though I don't know of any source for cold-pressed palm oil. You'll hear more about the benefits of coconut oil, in particular, later in this chapter.

Saturated fats can be a third to a half of your total fat intake, as long as they aren't hydrogenated or trans fats.

Trans Fat

Trans fats are formed when hydrogen is added to vegetable oil to convert it from a liquid to a solid (as in corn oil margarine, for example) in a process known as hydrogenation. This takes a potentially good polyunsaturated fat and fills it with protons, not only giving it an unhealthy positive charge but also rendering it useless in buffering acids. What's more, a structural change called cross linking occurs across the carbon chain of the fat that makes trans fats useless as metabolic fuel as well. And trans fats can interfere with optimal use of beneficial essential fatty acids (which we'll be getting to in a moment). You also get trans fats when heating polyunsaturated and monounsaturated fats above 118 degrees Fahrenheit. Any oil that isn't cold-pressed is going to have trans fats.

Trans fats raise cholesterol levels, impair circulation, and increase the risk of many degenerative diseases and age-related maladies. Trans fats are officially known as trans-fatty *acids*, which should give you a clue right there that they should have no place in your diet.

With no redeeming qualities, trans fat is the one type of fat you must avoid altogether. Following the pH Miracle Living plan, you won't find any trans fats in whole, natural foods—like the ones recommended in this book. Trans fats are the exclusive domain of processed foods, where they are used to extend the shelf life of foods, keeping them artificially "fresh" for extended periods. After the National Academy of Sciences published conclusions about the harmful health effects of trans fats in 2003, demonizing them more even than saturated fats, food labels began to note the amount of trans fats in some products. The FDA ruled in 2003 that food manufacturers must list trans fat amounts on nutrition labels, but the requirement doesn't go into effect until 2006. While you wait for access to more specific info, you can steer clear of trans fats by avoiding anything with "partially hydrogenated" or "vegetable shortening" in the list of ingredients. It pays to be scrupulous: Leading scientists at the Harvard School of Public Health estimate that 30,000 premature deaths every year are attributable to the consumption of trans-fatty acids.

Monounsaturated Fat

One of the wonderful properties of monounsaturated fats (besides their ability to cleanse the body of acids and fuel your metabolism) is that they are very stable. Unlike polyunsaturated fats (see below), they can withstand heat above 118 degrees F without breaking down into trans fats. That makes them the best choice when you cook your food.

Monounsaturated fats are usually liquid, though they will solidify in the refrigerator. The oils in olives and avocados are monounsaturated. Canola and peanut oils are also touted for being monounsaturated, but they are always processed with heat, which creates trans fats and so aren't good choices. "Cold-processed" oils are what you need; check the labels.

Polyunsaturated Fat

Electron-rich polyunsaturated fats can bind to more excess acids in the body than any other type of fat, and they are the best fuel for the body to use to generate energy. These fats will help lower your cholesterol levels because they buffer acids in your body, so less cholesterol is produced—and your risk of obesity is reduced, along with the risk of heart attack, stroke, and diabetes. In addition, the fats that are crucial in forming cell wall membranes are mainly polyunsaturated fats. If necessary, the body will use saturated fats for this purpose, but those membranes won't function as well as normal, which can lead to serious health problems over the long run.

Missing two or more pairs of hydrogen, polyunsaturated fats are found mainly in vegetable oils and are liquid at room temperature.

Polyunsaturated fats should make up 20 to 40 percent of your caloric intake—at least 60 to 90 grams of the stuff each day, for most people.

ESSENTIAL FATTY ACIDS: OMEGA-3 AND OMEGA-6

One subcategory of polyunsaturated fats are particularly . . . well, essential. The essential fatty acids (EFAs) are so called because the body needs but cannot make them; they must be provided via your food. There are two key groupings of EFAs I want to cover here: omega-3s and omega-6s, which are found in fish oils and a variety of seed oils. (Monounsaturated fats could be called omega-9s, though they rarely are.) These long-chain fats (18 to 22 carbon atoms in a row) are the very best acid neutralizers—big bus, plenty of open seats.

Omega-3s and omega-6s help build cell membranes, support the work of white blood cells, lubricate joints, insulate the body against heat loss, prevent skin from drying out, promote chromosome stability, improve brain function, enhance growth, improve lymphatic and blood circulation, support cellular growth and regeneration, and provide energy. They are used to make hormone-like prostaglandins that protect against heart disease, stroke, high blood pressure, atherosclerosis, blood clots, and diabetes. They can also help relieve secondary symptoms of arthritis, asthma, PMS, allergies, skin conditions, diabetes, and some behavior disorders. Deficiencies of omega-3s and omega-6s have been strongly implicated as a cause of serious disease—and obesity.

Mitzi

A lifetime of poor choices had left me tipping the scales at 240 pounds. I'd been up as high as 252. And I was sick enough with a variety of symptoms that I had been bedridden for just about two months. The only good thing about that condi-

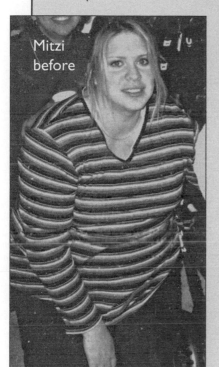

Mitzi
before

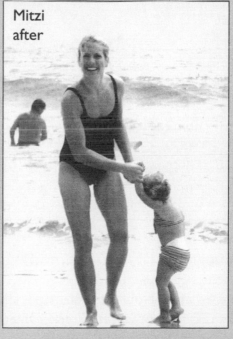

Mitzi
after

tion was that I had time to listen to my sister explain this program to me. It made sense to me from the start, and over time I studied up on the theory behind it in at least thirty different books. Finally, I decided to give it a try. I jumped in with both feet.

I threw away everything in my cabinets that was considered acidic and began drinking 5 to 6 green drinks a day. I went straight into a ten-day cleanse, which for me was highly uncomfortable—but apparently necessary. The more greens I drank, and the more days that passed without me indulging in acidic foods (or thoughts!), the stronger I could feel myself getting. Most of my health challenges, including migraines and extreme vertigo, disappeared. I am thrilled to say that **I lost 90 pounds in the first 90 days!** When I went to the gym to start training for a marathon, they measured my body fat to be at only 18 percent—and up to that point, I'd been doing no exercise. Almost two years later, I remain at a size 4–6 and love the simplicity of the program that keeps me at this size and in this state of health.

Bill

I started taking essential fats over seven years ago. While I initially took omega-3s for heart health, I discovered that a slightly larger dose helped me lose weight (30 pounds over nine months)—and maintain that weight loss.

Omega-3s: EPA, DHA, and ALA

The far end of the fat molecule is called the omega end, "omega" meaning final or last in Greek. Omega-3 fats are so called because the first missing pair of hydrogen atoms occurs at the third position from that end.

Omega-3s soak up the most acid of any kind of fat. That helps them decrease your risk of heart attack by lowering triglyceride levels (by as much as 65 percent) and cholesterol (especially LDL or "bad" cholesterol), reducing arteriosclerosis, lowering blood pressure, and improving blood circulation. A study at the Oregon Health Sciences University provided patients with high cholesterol and triglycerides omega-3s in the form of fish oil for four weeks—and their cholesterol dropped an average of 46 percent, and their triglycerides more than 75 percent! Omega-3s also reduce your risk of stroke.

In some animal studies, certain omega-3s even inhibited the growth and metastasis of tumors. That's probably because omega-3s help suppress formation of new blood supplies to tumors. In humans, this anticancer effect showed up in a French study documenting that women with high levels of a particular omega-3 (ALA) in the fat tissue in their breasts had a 60 percent lower risk of breast cancer than women with low levels, and Swedish studies showing men with high levels of omega-3s from fish oil in their blood had a lower risk of prostate cancer than men with low levels. Omega-3s fight inflammation, and so arthritis, colitis, fibromyalgia, diverticulitis, and other inflammatory diseases. They help prevent osteoporosis and diabetes. Last but certainly not least, omega-3 fats help keep you slim.

Two of the best sources of omega-3 fats are eicosapentaenoic acid (EPA) and docosahexaenoic acid (DHA), found in fatty cold water fish and other northern marine animals. Flaxseed, hemp, walnut, and soybean oils contain an omega-3 called alpha-linolenic acid (ALA), which the body converts, through several stages, into EPA then DHA. Flaxseed is the plant source richest in omega-3s, which comprise 57 percent of the oil. In addition, flaxseed oil contains about 16 percent omega-6s (see below).

EPA and DHA are abundant in brain cells, nerve relay stations, visual receptors, and adrenal and sex glands, to give you a feel for how integral they are in so many ways to the smooth functioning of the body.

Hayley

I have been using essential fats for five years. The combination of omega-3s and 6s helped me lose 35 pounds (prior to my wedding) and then quickly lose my "baby weight" after each of my two children were born. Plus, I know my two girls benefited from the good fats, too!

In 2000 the American Heart Association recommended that everyone should eat at least two 3-ounce servings of fatty fish each week. That same year even the FDA gave omega-3s its approval after reviewing evidence about reduction in risk of heart disease. In 2004, the FDA announced that it would allow products containing omega-3s to tout their heart-healthy benefits on the label and require specific information on how many grams of EPA or DHA are in the food.

Omega-6s: LA, CLA, and GLA

Omega-6 fats have their hydrogens missing in the sixth position away from the end of the chain. Though not quite up to the performance level of omega-3s, omega-6s are also good acid neutralizers and good to burn for energy. They help you burn off unwanted body fat by increasing your metabolic rate while you are burning fat for energy. Like omega-3s, omega-6s, too, help lower blood pressure, cholesterol levels, and risk of stroke and heart attack—and obesity. Not to mention helping prevent arthritis, stop cancer cells, improve diabetic side effects, relieve PMS, and improve the condition of hair, nails, and skin.

The two key omega-6 fats are linoleic acid (LA) and gamma-linolenic acid (GLA). Omega-6s are readily available in your diet, since they occur in a range of common vegetable oils, nuts, and seeds. In addition, omega-6s are made from omega-3s within the body as they soak up protons. LA is found in safflower, soybean, sesame, walnut, pumpkin, flax, and hemp—seeds, nuts, and oils. LA and GLA are both found in sunflower, evening primrose, black currant, and borage oils. The amount contained varies by the oil, and most oils have a combination of omega-6s. Borage seed oil, for example, contains up to 24 percent GLA—more than twice the level in evening primrose oil—and about 34 percent LA.

Studies at the Welsh National School of Medicine have shown that GLA from evening primrose and borage oils stimulates the metabolism and so increases fat burning. In one study, participants lost an average of about 10 pounds over a six-week period when they

Antonia

For most of my life, I have been consumed in a search for the right diet. Food has always been a focal point of my life, the aromas of home-cooked meals and the large quantities of food prepared for gatherings with family and friends—the sheer enjoy-

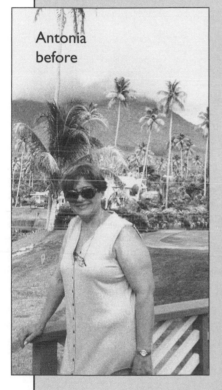

Antonia before

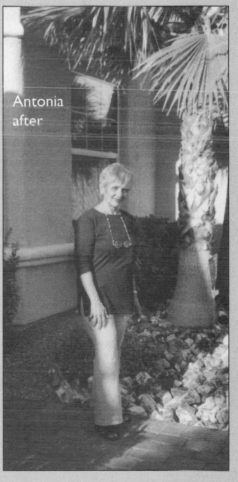

Antonia after

ment of a good meal. My wardrobe consisted of "fat clothes" and "not-so-fat" clothes. As my waistline expanded, so did my repertoire of diet plans. I even experimented with diet pills. I was on a vicious cycle that was controlling my life and literally driving me crazy.

After years of this madness, I knew I could no longer continue on this path but, having tried just about everything, didn't know where else to turn. The turning point in my life came when my husband became seriously ill with cancer, slowly deteriorating before my eyes. It was a horrible experience and one that I will never forget. His death had a profound effect on me, as I realized I certainly never wanted to live through something like that, and I didn't want to put anyone else through it. I promised myself that for the sake of myself and my children, I would no longer concentrate on losing weight. Instead, I decided to focus on getting and staying healthy. Seeing how this program had helped my daughter, I started to incorporate it into my own life. I began transitioning slowly, faithfully drinking green drink while adjusting my lifestyle and eating habits. I learned to prepare healthy meals that were both delicious and satisfying. To my surprise, my cravings began to subside, I found new energy, my skin began clearing up, and, as an extra perk, the excess weight started to melt away! I'm now 45 pounds lighter and have found that it is easy for me to maintain my weight. I feel better and look better. I have regained youth and vitality, and I am proud to say that as I am about to celebrate my seventieth birthday, I feel more like forty!

took GLA. Animal studies conducted at the National Food Research Institute in Japan demonstrated that when taking GLA from borage oil, less body fat accumulates.

A form of LA called conjugated linoleic acid, or CLA, reduces the body's ability to store fat and promotes the use of stored fat for energy. A study published in the *Journal of Nutrition* in 2000 found a 20 percent decrease in body fat percentage and an average loss of 7 pounds of fat over a ninety-day period in patients taking CLA and *not* making any changes to their diets. The study compared different doses of CLA against placebo and found that 3.54 grams (g) of CLA per day was sufficient to obtain all the beneficial effects.

A Norwegian study published in 2001 in the *Journal of International Medical Research* demonstrated that CLA helped people exercising strenuously three times a week significantly reduce their body fat and increase lean muscle mass compared to those following the exercise program but not taking CLA. Neither group made any other changes to their lifestyle during the trial.

EAT FAT

Inuits in Greenland eat more fat than any other people in the world. Yet heart disease, strokes, and cancer are virtually unknown among them. Their secret: omega-3 fats. Because their diet is so heavily based on fish and northern marine animals, omega-3s make up 10 percent of their total blood fats. (For comparison's sake, a study of Danes living in Copenhagen following essentially the same diet as the typical American one showed almost no omega-3s in their blood. My own studies show the typical American's levels are less than 3 percent.) Just imagine what a similar level of omega-3s could do for you, especially combined with the rich plant nutrition of the pH Miracle Living plan.

Eating fat—the right fat—will *lower* your cholesterol and blood pressure, and *reduce* the plaque in your arteries, despite whatever the many fat-phobes out there may say. Thus, one of the many points of this plan is to increase the amount of healthy, electron-rich mono- and polyunsaturated fats, and even saturated fats, in your diet. That means virgin, cold-pressed, or low heat–extracted oils like olive, flaxseed, borage, and primrose. It also means fish, especially trout, salmon, mackerel, sardines, tuna, striped bass, and eel, the richest sources of EPA and DHA omega-3s. And it means foods that contain naturally occurring oils. Fish is one example, and nuts and seeds are also generally rich in healthy fats. Here I want to call attention to two other key foods in particular: avocado and coconut.

Avocado is a key source of monounsaturated fats in the pH Miracle Living plan, right up there with olive oil, and you should have at least one a day—up to three to five for those with serious health conditions. Avocados are important in reaching and maintaining your ideal weight because they neutralize acids, protecting your body against the inevitable by-products of digestion, metabolism, and respiration. That's job one in the fight against obesity. And like other monounsaturated fats, avocado helps protect the heart and blood vessels. Avocados contain compounds that lower cholesterol and help prevent certain types of cancers, eye disease, heart disease, diabetes, and obesity—in greater concentrations than many other commonly eaten plant foods. Avocados have antioxidant as well as antacid properties. They contain fourteen minerals, notably iron and copper, which aid in red blood cell regeneration, and potassium. They are one of the best sources of vitamin E. They contain no starch and very little sugar. Avocados are 80 percent fat, all of it good. And they are a good source of protein (10 to 15 percent). (To buy organic avocados via mail order, see Resources.)

Coconut is the second incredible fat-rich food you should never do without when you are working toward a healthy weight. Technically a saturated fat, coconut oil—as long as it is cold pressed and not converted into trans fat by heat processing—has been shown to reduce the symptoms of digestive disorders, support the work of the white blood cells, and help prevent bacterial, yeast, and fungal infections. Coconut oil is high in lauric fats (which comprise 50 to 55 percent of its makeup), a medium-chain fat that the body converts into monolaurin. Monolaurin helps reduce acidity and, thus, weight. By controlling yeast, coconut oil reduces yeast's appetite—and your cravings for sugar. It also curbs hypoglycemia and helps eliminate hunger pangs. The final bit of good news about coconut: It speeds up your metabolism. A study conducted in Yucatan, where coconut is a staple of the diet, showed that people living there had metabolic rates 25 percent higher than people with a similar profile living in the United States. (Bonus: The women in Yucatan had none of the symptoms commonly associated with menopause.)

You'll get more details on how to work good fats into your foods on the pH Miracle Living plan in chapter 12. Basically, I recommend increasing your omega-3s, 6s, and 9s by eating wild (not farm-raised) salmon, mackerel, trout, tuna, striped bass, and other cold-water fish several times a week. You should also include flax oil and Essential Oil by Braleans on steamed veggies or in soups, shakes, and salad dressings every day. To increase your omega-6s, also use oils from hemp, primrose, and borage. And eat almonds, hazelnuts, flax, and sunflower seeds—raw, not roasted. Get a variety of oils in your diet. In every case, select unrefined, cold-pressed organic oils (check your local natural food store). Exposure to heat, light, and even oxygen makes fats and oils rancid, which, besides affecting their taste, reduces their beneficial properties. So choose oils in dark containers to protect them from light exposure, and buy smaller bottles to reduce exposure to air. Check the selections in the refrigerator section of your natural food store. Leave out enough oil for a few days' use, and freeze the rest to extend the life of the oil you've invested in. Yes, high-quality oils will be more expensive, but the good health they provide is priceless.

The following chart summarizes the best sources of fats. In addition, I recommend supplementing your good fats intake. You'll find the details of the pH Miracle Living plan in chapter 12.

Good Fats and Where to Find Them

Most oils contain both monounsaturated and polyunsaturated fats, and are generally classified by which one makes up the greater proportion. Again make sure to buy cold-pressed oils; heating the oil during extraction and/or packaging breaks it down, robbing it of its benefits.

GOOD Saturated fats for energy	BETTER Monounsaturated fats for acid buffering	BEST Polyunsaturated fats for acid buffering and cellular membranes	
		Omega-3s	Omega-6s
coconut oil	olive oil	marine oils	borage oil
	cold-pressed canola oil	fish oils	evening primrose oil
	almond oil	flaxseeds and oil	soybean oil
	avocado and avocado oil	hemp oil	sesame oil
	raw nuts		sesame seeds and oil
			safflower oil
			pumpkin seeds
			black currant oil
			sunflower oil
			grapeseed oil

Used on a regular basis, electron-rich fats provide many health benefits and are especially important to reaching your ideal weight. A 2000 report from the Surgeon General on nutrition and health declares that deficiencies, excesses, or imbalances of fat in the body are involved in 70 percent or more of all deaths in this country. Choose the right fats, get plenty of them, and you'll never be one of those statistics. You'll stick at your ideal weight, in vibrant good health besides.

Chapter 7

Think Thin

*If you don't consciously prepare yourself each day to practice wonder
and joy, you get really good at practicing stress and pain and
anger and anxiety and fear . . . kids laugh 300 to 400
times a day. But grown-ups? Only about 15.*
—SARANNE ROTHBERG, founder of Comedy Cures

Thoughts and emotions—your mental, psychological, emotional, and
even spiritual state—can actually make your body more—or less—
acidic. Similarly, what you eat can affect your thoughts, moods, and
emotions. Eating the wrong kinds of foods can lead to depression—
and overeating. Eat the right kinds of foods brings a feeling of overall well-being and even euphoria. This chapter is designed to help
you make sure your mind works for you, not against you, when it
comes to weight loss.

Behavior is complex, and so is changing it. There is no quick fix.
But understanding how our thoughts and feelings in general, and
about food in particular, influence us and our lifestyle choices is critical to not just getting to a healthy weight, but also staying there.
You need an attitude that will help you on your way, as well as specific tools to help you move ahead positively.

THINK POSITIVE

For the body to stay in a healthy state of balance, including a healthy weight, you must find mental, emotional, and spiritual calm, as well as physical stability. Our thoughts and emotions can disturb the balance just as more obvious physical challenges can, leading to the excess acidity in the body at the root of excess weight. This book would be unfinished if we left it at "you are what you eat—and drink." You are also what you think. Being stuck in negative thoughts and emotions will contribute to trapping you in an acidic, overweight body—you're actually thinking yourself fat. Finding an emotional balance and a sense of spiritual connection, on the other hand, you can actually think yourself thin.

On a very basic level, uncontrolled negative thoughts and emotions often trigger unhealthy eating in a variety of forms, aimed at comforting and consoling oneself. We often overeat under stress, or eat when we're nervous, or eat for a momentary good feeling, or eat because we are lonely, or eat to reward ourselves, or eat to fill a void, or eat to punish ourselves for being unhappy—and so on, and so on. And we may choose unhealthy foods because we are feeling generally negative, or because they remind us of happy childhood memories. Obviously, these eating binges, whatever their particulars, overtax the body, especially since they almost always entail sugar, carbs, and/or too much protein. Then, as we pack on more fat and/or unhealthy eating, our thoughts and feelings just go downhill, creating a vicious cycle. As you spiral around, you're liable to just give up, to stop even trying to improve your health.

To change only your diet isn't enough to achieve permanent weight loss and vibrant good health. You must also deal with any emotional issues and stresses by understanding and modifying your behavior. Leaving them out of control will undermine even the best of intentions about what you eat. We all need to find ways to think and feel differently, to use negative thoughts and emotions in constructive ways rather than wallowing in them, and we need to do that even when we are under stress.

I (Shelley) am certainly not advising you to not be emotional. That's simply not humanly possible, anyway. Being human means having emotions. It's not enough to tell yourself just to not think negatively, or to *get over it* or *not be upset*. That will never last, if it ever works. Just as the basic principles of diet and exercise need to be learned, understood, considered, accepted, and adopted, so too do you need to process your thoughts and emotions as well as your approach to them. That begins by recognizing that your emotions come from your thoughts, and those thoughts from your beliefs.

Our beliefs give rise to our thoughts and to our behavior. That is to say, our beliefs are the foundation upon which we build our very selves. Our worldview, our values and judgments, impact all of our decisions and the way we relate to others.

Our thoughts are our constant companions, so it's no wonder they are so integral to our overall health. Thoughts can lift you up when they form dreams, bring joy, or recall happy memories, or drag you down when they present fear, suspicion, and worry. Thoughts can keep us stuck in past or future moments, distracting us from living in the present, engaging whatever is in front of us at the current moment. Thoughts can be true or false, and they are powerful either way. In order for our thoughts to contribute to sound health and permanent weight loss, they must add to our sense of well-being, fulfill our needs, and not add any undue amount of anxiety or stress. Learning to understand, handle, and control your thoughts as they happen to you will prevent an accumulation of negative emotions and help you develop supportive behavior patterns conducive to healthy living, including nourishing yourself properly.

Emotions, too, can be positive or negative. In his book *Power Vs. Force* Dr. David R. Hawkins rates the energy level of basic human emotions on a scale of 1 to 1,000, stating that anything hitting 200 or lower will be destructive of life both for the individual and for the society, while anything above that level represents constructive expressions of power. Here's his rankings:

Shame	20
Guilt	30
Apathy	50
Grief	75
Fear	100

Desire	125
Anger	150
Pride	175
Courage	200
Neutrality (no judgment)	250
Willingness	310
Acceptance	350
Reason	400
Love	500
Joy	540
Peace	600
Enlightenment	700–1,000

You'll want to live your life, of course, among the higher-ranking feelings on Dr. Hawkins' scale. Your sense of self and well-being is best served by healthy emotions and positive thoughts. When bad things happen, it's realistic to experience difficult emotional seasons, but it helps to have your inner compass set when you are ready to move on. You need to experience your feelings fully, but not linger too long in negative ones that could leave you physically imbalanced as well. You'll need to call on many approaches to alleviate negative emotions and prevent them from getting a strong hold on your body, including resolve, forgiveness, restitution, and reconciliation.

SPIRITUALITY

The true source of well-being, joy, and contentment lies within one's own mind and heart and not in the physical world. You may be trying to find that place by controlling your physical body—losing weight and getting healthy—but the truth is you need to find that place first, to allow the physical changes to come easily.

That's why you need to embrace a more spiritual vision of yourself and of humanity as a whole. That's the way to live and work and love with less fear and stress. Most of us live in two worlds: the world of doing and the world of being. The world of doing is generally concerned with making our lives and the lives of our loved ones more comfortable, trying to fulfill our needs, desires, longings, expectations, identity, and cultural conditioning. This road rarely leads to genuine happiness or a connection to our emotional and spiritual selves. When one problem is solved, another one appears. When one goal is achieved, it is only a matter of time before another one shows up and we are chasing after a new pursuit.

The world of being lies deep within all of us. It is our true self, our spiritual nature. It is characterized by silence, stillness, freedom, and love. Living in this world helps us to be calm. It puts us back in touch with what we value most: fairness, kindness, forgiveness, compassion, hope, love, and charity. Here the focus shifts from the physical world of what should be *done* (including about your health or weight) to the timeless, dimensionless part of one's inner spiritual self that is already vibrantly healthy and does not need to *do* anything—just be.

BELIEVE IN THE pH MIRACLE

Step 1 for channeling your inner life positively is to believe in the approach to health you choose. In this instance, that means full faith in the alkaline approach as the very best we can do for ourselves and our bodies. A miracle requires faith! They key is to accept and practice the pH Miracle Living program not as restrictive, or a form of deprivation, but as rich and abundantly full of foods most suited to supporting ideal weight and health. Healthy foods are a blessing available to us, and with that in mind we can feel a sense of gratitude—a positive emotion—for the undertaking. And the more we eat the foods that are best for us, the more peaceful our minds will be.

So how we think about how we care for ourselves determines not only how likely we are to adhere to the lifestyle we choose, but also how much we will get out of it. That's why we think it is so important for you to understand the principles behind each of our recommendations. I could write just one page of instructions for you to follow and leave it at that, but I don't think you'd be able to put much stock in that without a full explanation of the rhyme and reason of it all. And the more you get out of the program, the stronger your belief in its rightness will be.

As your belief grows stronger, the alkaline lifestyle will become pretty much second nature to you; you'll eventually follow it more or less automatically. That's important to remember as you are starting out, when it seems there is so much to absorb. It can seem overwhelming. But don't let that (temporary!) feeling prevent you from pursuing this solution to finding—and living at—your ideal weight. This is not a "diet" to go on and off of, it is a lifetime plan.

You will only be able to change your behavior after you have your beliefs, thoughts, and emotions where you want them to be. Once you do, it will be easy to decide what to put on your plate and in your mouth.

Make Sure Your Beliefs Are True

One important stop on the journey to thinking yourself thin is to recognize any false beliefs you might hold and correct them. If you don't, false thoughts will follow, with negative emotions in tow. For example, you may believe that fat is bad, ugly, a sign of weakness, or a punishment, and because of that *you* think you are bad, ugly, weak, and deserve punishment. You may believe that being fat is genetic and that if your parents are fat your fate is pretty much sealed. You may believe you can put responsibility for your weight on some one or some thing other than yourself—your partner, a weight-loss expert, some magic bullet pill. You may believe that the best way to choose your food is by what pleases your taste buds most, or by what is most readily available.

Leaving those beliefs, or any others like them, behind you leaves your path to your ideal weight clear. Recognizing, for example, that rather than being bad, your fat has actually been saving your life—to this point—lets you think differently about its accumulation on your hips, stomach, thighs, and so forth. You can *love* your fat, *thank* it for protecting your health—and then, with your new awareness and alkaline lifestyle, *say good-bye* to it. Forever. After all, you'll no longer need it.

On the pH Miracle Living plan, "dieting" is no longer about pure willpower, but rather comprises a new behavior coming as a result of a changed belief, thought, and, perhaps, emotion. Your new understanding of weight, fat, and health lets you make good food choices, acting on the principles of the pH Miracle. Your thinking becomes something like, "I choose my foods and drinks according to what I believe will be best for my health, energy, and emotional well-being. I give myself the very best delicious, alkalizing food on the planet because I know this food will keep me at my ideal weight and health." Eating well becomes the great reward in life—not that brownie or that steak!

Once you are thinking intelligently about your food choices ("If I eat acid, I will gain weight; if I eat alkaline, I will lose weight or stay at my ideal weight"), and working with true and positive emotions, especially surrounding your health and weight, you'll be able to really put the principles of the pH Miracle into practice. And following the principles will ensure your ideal weight.

How to Think Thin
- Avoid unnecessary emotional stress in your life.
- Develop strategies to handle unavoidable stress efficiently and constructively, and quickly move on.
- Learn to act upon, not *react* to, whatever you may face. Take a step back from the situation, and view it objectively, without judgment, moving away from the *feel* of any negative emotion.
- Stay in the present.
- Do not linger in negative thoughts or emotions.
- Stay positive.
- Don't beat yourself up if you slip up. Forgive yourself, and keep going.
- Avoid the accumulation of negative thoughts or emotions.
- Expect that you (like everyone else) will go through several emotions on any given day—and that some will be positive and some will be negative. Practice facing those emotions

head-on, solving problems quickly if possible, changing false beliefs and destructive negative emotional reactions—and reserving your energy for more enjoyable, relaxed times.

- Discover how your emotions relate to your eating habits. Don't use eating as a coping mechanism. Learn other, more productive ways to cope.
- Get plenty of rest. A good night's sleep is vital to a normal metabolism. Insomnia, or waking up at 2 or 3 A.M., many times results from an emotional issue surfacing in your subconscious and disturbing restful sleep. It can also be related to adrenal exhaustion from a stress.
- If necessary, or if you find yourself repeatedly "falling off the wagon," consider consulting a therapist to help you unlock pent-up emotional issues and resolve them.
- Set realistic short- and long-term goals and have reasonable expectations of yourself. Value your weight-loss process and goal. How much do you desire to be slim and healthy again?
- Give yourself a realistic time frame or deadline, and commit to it.
- Reward yourself without food. As you reach your goals, give yourself a huge pat on the back—and continue on. Choose as rewards something you value, like signing up for a class you've always wanted to take, going on a trip, shopping for a new outfit in a smaller size, or treating yourself to a piece of art to hang in your home (every time you pass it, you'll be reminded of your accomplishment).
- Take time every day for contemplation, prayer, or meditation. Realize all your blessings and express your gratitude.
- Discover what triggers you to eat what's not good for you—stress, comfort, socializing—and seek to avoid them. You need to understand your urges in order to manage them.
- Express your emotions. Laugh. Cry.
- Believe in yourself.
- Work on your own self-interest. Make time and space to do what's best for you; do what will make you healthy, strong, smart—and happy. That applies well beyond the realm of

Scott

I've lost weight before. But I always fell off the wagon and regained it, especially when trying to help others do what I had done when they weren't ready for a change. On this program, I just focused on creating balance for myself, studied the books aggressively, and committed myself 100 percent. I have not had meat, dairy, eggs, bread, or sugar for nine weeks now—and I've lost 40 pounds!

With all the lemons, limes, tomatoes, almonds, and avocados on my plate, I don't even crave the foods I've cut out. I love experimenting with Shelley's great recipes. I even invented my own salad dressing!

Several chronic health problems have cleared up. I'm thinking sharper, concentrating better, and not sleeping twelve to fourteen hours a day like I used to. Now, six or seven hours of sleep is plenty. I've been able to get all those house projects done that I had been putting off for years! I let go of my negative thoughts, words, and deeds. My friends see a difference in me. Some of them are even learning about the importance of vegetables and alkaline foods.

food. Go back to school, take an art class, dare to dream—and then do it.
- Think about weight loss not as an event but as a journey. Make it a new and exciting growth experience. Be grateful for all you'll learn along the way.

THE CHOICE IS YOURS

The ultimate key to all of this is you. You have to decide that you are going to change for the better. No one can make this choice for you, nor can you put responsibility on anyone else. No plan works without you doing your part. If you want to be your ideal weight, if you want health, energy, vitality, you have to do it. You can't buy it or get it ready-made. You are free to choose, right or wrong. You can eat salad or steak. You can drink good water or not. You can commit to exercising or not. You can be slim or not. The choice is yours.

While you choose, you should keep in mind that the choices you are making have an impact not only on you, but also on your family, community, and society.

MAP YOUR ROUTE

The journey to success involves asking yourself where you are, where you're going, and how you're going to get there. There's no other way to find the right path for yourself—and stay on it. If you don't like where you've been, or where you are, clearly you're going to have to change tracks!

To move forward in the best direction, start by clarifying your destination. That is, set your goal. You need something specific (and measurable) to aim for. Otherwise, how will you know when or if you get there? Your goal also needs to be reasonable; planning to shed fifteen years' worth of excess weight, and at least as many years' worth of bad habits with lightning speed is only setting yourself up for failure. Your goal also needs to have a time frame. So, decide you want to lose 20 pounds by June, and be at your ideal weight of 145 pounds by August. Or that you want to lower your blood pressure to within normal range within three months. Or that you want to wear a size 8 dress to the annual Christmas party. Or that you want to put on 10 pounds' worth of muscle. Think carefully about exactly what you are after. Then, write it down. Committing it to paper is how you commit yourself to it.

Break it down, now. You've got your final destination in mind and your overall goal, and now you need to plot out the specific stops on your trip. These should be smaller markers you can keep an eye on to make sure you are still going in the right direction: changing one thing about your diet each week, or cutting back on portion size, or buying more fresh produce. Once again, write down your plan.

HOW MUCH SHOULD I WEIGH?

Setting weight-loss goals can be tricky. Aim for too much and you risk discouragement. Aim for too little and you won't claim the fullest good health. And getting to the same size you were in high school, or fitting into the jeans you wore before you got pregnant the first time, may never happen for you—the healthiest size and shape for you this much further down the line might just be different, even though you will be lean and fit.

I recommend finding your range of healthy weight using the body mass index (BMI), which describes body weight relative to height and is strongly correlated with body fat content in adults. Start by looking up your height and weight on the following chart. If your BMI comes out higher than 25, that's considered overweight, and your risk of various unpleasant effects (like heart disease, and death) rises. Above 30 is considered obese, and above 40 extremely obese, and your risks just keep increasing.

Aim to get your weight into the normal zone for your height, whatever would give you a BMI under 25. (Less than 18.5 is *under*weight and you don't want to go there any more than you want to go over.)

You might want to fine tune your BMI expectations for yourself by taking your waist measurement into account. Excess abdominal fat—of which your waist measurement is a strong indicator—is also associated with increased risk of disease and death. A waist measuring over 40 inches in men, or 35 inches in women, increases the risk further still for those with BMIs between 25 and 35. You should aim to get your belt size under that threshold. For some people that might require getting their BMI into the lower range of normal, rather than the upper.

BMI (kg/m^2)	19	20	21	22	23	24	25	26	27	28	29	30	35	40
Height (in.)							Weight (lbs.)							
58	91	96	100	105	110	115	119	124	129	134	138	143	167	191
59	94	99	104	109	114	119	124	128	133	138	143	148	173	198
60	97	102	107	112	118	123	128	133	138	143	148	153	179	204
61	100	106	111	116	122	127	132	137	143	148	153	158	185	211
62	104	109	115	120	126	131	136	142	147	153	158	164	191	218
63	107	113	118	124	130	135	141	146	152	158	163	169	197	225
64	110	116	122	128	134	140	145	151	157	163	169	174	204	232
65	114	120	126	132	138	144	150	156	162	168	174	180	210	240
66	118	124	130	136	142	148	155	161	167	173	179	186	216	247
67	121	127	134	140	146	153	159	166	172	178	185	191	223	255
68	125	131	138	144	151	158	164	171	177	184	190	197	230	262
69	128	135	142	149	155	162	169	176	182	189	196	203	236	270
70	132	139	146	153	160	167	174	181	188	195	202	207	243	278
71	136	143	150	157	165	172	179	186	193	200	208	215	250	286
72	140	147	154	162	169	177	184	191	199	206	213	221	258	294
73	144	151	159	166	174	182	189	197	204	212	219	227	265	302
74	148	155	163	171	179	186	194	202	210	218	225	233	272	311
75	152	160	168	176	184	192	200	208	216	224	232	240	279	319
76	156	164	172	180	189	197	205	213	221	230	238	246	287	328

BMI	
18.5 or less	Underweight
18.5–24.9	Normal
25.0–29.9	Overweight
30.0–39.9	Obese
40 or more	Extremely Obese

Keep in mind that you set the pace. Your progress will depend on your commitment and effort, but also on your goal, your starting point, and the path you plan to take from one to the other. I've seen clients who totally alkalize their diet and drink 5 or 6 liters a day of green drink (more on green drink later) from the get-go, and drop as much as 90 pounds in 90 days. And I've seen other clients who hydrate properly, with greens sometimes, yet still have the occasionally acidic food, and lose less weight over a longer period of time.

Asherah

I've spent thousands of dollars and tried many different health and weight-loss programs over the past fifteen years, but nothing really worked. I was overweight and had been plagued for years by chronic health challenges. Until this program changed my life forever. When I had live blood analysis done, I discovered my blood was full of yeast and the toxins from yeast, and that really got me focused on making some

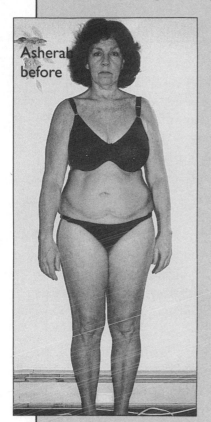

Asherah before

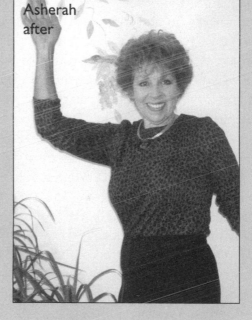

Asherah after

changes, and taking my life and my health into my own hands.

For the first two weeks after I started using the green drink, I lost a pound a day—and I hadn't made any changes to my diet. I was so amazed I decided to do the full program, starting with a cleanse and then eating alkaline foods from Shelley's recipes. I lost 35 pounds in eight weeks and watched the cellulite disappear from my thighs. At fifty-nine years old I am looking younger and feeling more energetic than I have since I was in my thirties.

Now ask yourself—and note down your most detailed and honest answers—*why* you want what you want. Broaden your scope again, as far as you can. In the service of what, exactly, do you want to lose that 20 pounds or buy new clothes? What is your purpose on this journey? Is your ultimate aim to feel good? Look good? Feel good about yourself? Feel in control of your life? Increase your strength? Have more energy? Raise your self-esteem? Live longer? Feel sexy? Be healthy?

There's no one right answer. In fact, there's not just one answer for any given person. But it always pays to know why you want whatever you're after. Once you know why you want something, the how is not so hard. Once you are clear on your reasons, you can move forward without hesitation. A compelling purpose gives you the drive to follow through.

Now you're ready to get down to the nitty-gritty of creating an action plan for yourself—and writing it down. And I don't just mean scribbling "follow the pH Miracle Living program." You need to lay out exactly what you're going to do and when and how. That means, planning a time to go produce shopping at least once a week; getting to know your local health food store and especially the oils and supplements therein; cutting out all acidic foods immediately; taking a more gradual approach by eliminating dessert this week, pasta next week, and so on; and making dates with yourself for exercising. Take stock of the resources available to you as you progress: the people, places, and things that can help you get where you want to go, like a like-minded friend, the gym, or a rebounder—then put them to work. Be sure to build in some flexibility to make sure your specific plan is doable for you in your busy life.

There are many ways to achieve a result, so as long as you stay focused on what you want, have a strong purpose to drive you, and stay flexible in your approach, you will find your way.

JOURNAL

As you've seen, you're going to need to be doing a lot of writing. As a human being, you're bound to forget about even important things within three to five days if you are not constantly reminded of them. So if you haven't done it already, I recommend starting a private journal to not only keep track of the specifics of your progress, as in chapter 11, but also your mental and emotional journey.

In addition to the things I've asked you to write down over the course of this chapter already, here are some other topics that should get your pen moving: Do you really want to lose weight and get healthy? How will it make you feel to accomplish your goal? What will you gain if you do? What will you lose (besides pounds!)? How will getting healthy and slim affect your everyday life, both in the short term and long term? How will your life be affected if you fail? Do you believe you can succeed? How committed are you to your goal, and to your plan for reaching it? Do you feel you deserve to be healthy and fit?

Your journal should help you through the actual weight-loss process. You can use it to track the details of your progress, your measurements, and so on. I recommend keeping a food diary, taking notes on what you eat and where and why (your mood at the time). Review it every so often, not just to see if you are making smart food choices, but also to see if you can pinpoint a pattern to when you make bad choices. If you are using food to soothe or reward yourself, for example, look for healthier alternatives.

Furthermore, your journal should help make sure your thoughts, emotions, beliefs, and spirit are ready and willing to support you along the way. Write down both physical and emotional challenges. Spend some time with your journal every day—if not writing in it, then reviewing the wealth of information and inspiration already in there. Or both! It will only help to constantly review what you want to be, what you want to attain. Seeing the reasons you've documented for your weight-loss journey will boost your motivation.

JUST BEGIN

The hardest part is to begin. Once you do get started, it will get easier every day to follow this program. As you begin to practice the principles in this book, and in this chapter, you'll be able to see the changes that occur as a result, on the physical, psychological, and spiritual levels. As you begin feeling (and looking!) better, you'll start thinking better, and when you are thinking better, you will also do better. Not only will the weight start to come off, but also you'll experience more energy, feel less pain, be less sick, and generally feel a sense of overall well-being. All this will confirm for you that you are on the right path.

If you fall off the wagon once in a while, just hop right back on. The more you stay on, the less you'll fall off. Weight loss is not a single event, it is a process. You have to take it one step at a time. It may not be easy, but it's worth it. *You* are worth it.

Chapter 8

Eat Right for Your Life

*Food is a sacrament, never trivial—a view that sheds new light on
how you eat. Your earthly body won't be around forever. For more
energy here, forge an intuitive partnership with the fuel you feed it.
Such cooperation with diet and in all areas, increases your life force,
which wants you to be vibrant. Expect results. The positive changes
that come from an energy-aware diet are proof of success.*
—Judith Orloff, M.D.

The human body takes in an average of 5½ pounds of food and
drink each day. That amounts to 1 ton of solid and liquid nourish-
ment annually. Over the course of seventy years, an average person
eats and drinks about 1,000 times his or her weight. At that kind of
volume, no wonder exactly what we put into our mouths—into our
bodies—is so important.

So far, we've not been choosing too well. For one thing, our
choices have made us extremely fat, and these choices have raised
our risk of a huge range of health problems, many of them deadly.
For another, the average American diet has suboptimal levels of a
wide range of nutrients; while we may get enough to avoid deficiency syndromes, we get so little of so many critical nutrients as to
increase our risk further still for many chronic diseases. Although in
some cases supplements may be the key to ensuring your body gets
exactly what it needs (see chapter 9), the best defense is eating right.
The huge number of biological, active compounds in all foods,
which interact in complex ways with each other and with the body,
means supplementation cannot substitute for good food.

The eating plan in this book puts us on the right path once again, so we can enjoy lean, strong, healthy bodies. This chapter describes the best diet for permanent weight loss [low-protein, low-carb, high (good) fats—and veggies galore]. It gives you the specific alkaline foods to eat and drink and acidic foods to avoid, and presents the "house of health™" plan for eating in a pH-balanced way.

Generally speaking, you'll get and stay slim and healthy on a diet that is relatively low in carbs and protein; rich in good, healthy fats; and focused around a wide variety of green vegetables. You should eat whole, natural, unprocessed organic foods. Processed and fast foods are all acidic, as are canned, fried, and microwaved foods. And you want a clear majority of your food to be truly alive. Live (raw)

FAST FOOD: MAKING YOU FAT, FAST

The filmmaker Morgan Spurlock shocked audiences at the 2004 Sundance Film Festival with *Super Size Me,* which chronicled his thirty-day diet of eating nothing but food from McDonald's. He gained 25 pounds, his cholesterol shot up— and his liver began to fail. But we didn't really need Mr. Spurlock to tell us all this, did we? We already know the tidal wave of American obesity is intimately linked with fast foods.

Shortly after the release of Mr. Spurlock's movie, McDonald's announced they were downsizing and doing away with their Super Size fries and drinks by the end of the year. But I don't believe for one moment that reducing the size of the servings will reduce the waistlines of America. You might be getting less of it, but it will still be acidic through and through. If we dine on proton-rich acidic food like that, we will never be satisfied because we aren't providing the body what it really needs, and we'll end up eating five times as much food as we need. It is only with electron-rich alkaline food that the body really gets what it needs, and what will satisfy it.

food is electron-rich. All this will keep your body alkaline, which will keep you healthy—and at your ideal weight.

YOUR ENERGY BANK ACCOUNT

Think of your body as a bank account. When you eat electron-rich alkaline food, you are making a deposit to your account, maintaining an investment in your health, fitness, energy, vitality—and weight. And when you eat proton-saturated acidic food, you are making an energy withdrawal. On the most basic level, if there's not enough in the account to cover withdrawals, you're in trouble! If you withdraw too much, your body has to struggle to maintain a positive balance (pH balance). When your account is completely depleted of electrons, you are dead! To keep a good balance, so you always have enough energy on hand to draw on as necessary, you need to both limit your withdrawals and make plenty of deposits (in the form of green foods, green drinks, and good fats). We'll get to the kinds of things that take electrons out of your account, but first we'll begin with your best bets when it comes to deposits.

Ginger

On my forty-eighth birthday, I decided I was sick and tired of being sick and tired, sick and tired of being on so many medications, and sick and tired of being fat—and that I was finally going to institute some real change in my life, and get healthy. I jumped into the pH Miracle program with both feet, and I never looked back.

I lost 20 pounds in the first twelve days. After two months, I was down 35 pounds, to my ideal weight.

My diet isn't perfectly alkaline yet, but the changes I've made in how I eat have already brought wonderful results. I have green drink, which I affectionately call my "swamp grass water," at least three times a day, including for breakfast. I'm not that hungry at lunch, so I usually have some raw and steamed vegetables, or hummus and chips, with some soymilk. For supper—my favorite meal!—I always have a huge salad (I have about six combinations I like to rotate through so I don't get bored), sometimes with a little chicken, shrimp, or tofu. I make spaghetti, chili, fresh fish, new potatoes, veggie pizza—the list is endless, but I make sure to start with a really big salad before I eat a small serving of those as side dishes. Sometimes, I still treat myself to soy ice cream or sesame cookies. I even eat out a lot; every place has a great salad!

I have lost my appetite for meat, wheat, sugar, and pop. I drink only distilled water—a gallon a day. And I exercise for forty-five minutes three times a week besides walking at least an hour a day—and push-mowing the lawn.

Besides the thrill of losing all that weight—and with no sagging skin left behind—I drastically reduced the amount of insulin I need, and, along with my doctor's help, weaned myself off several other medications as well. I no longer take over-the-counter vitamins. Who needs them when I have my greens?! I also need much less sleep than before, though I always have way more energy than I used to.

It hasn't exactly been a breeze, but it hasn't been that hard, either. I believe in this program, in part because it is always simple (even when it isn't always easy). And whatever it takes, it is more than worth it to me to be healthy, happy—and gorgeous!

Alkaline Foods

The heart of this plan are the electron-rich green foods and drinks and healthy fats, and you can eat them freely. This gives you a huge spectrum of wonderful foods to choose from, and toward the end of this chapter you'll find a more comprehensive listing of them. Here I'm going to take the time and space to detail only the most important of them.

Essential Fatty Acids

Chapter 6 details the benefits of good fats, so here I'd just like to recommend a few foods rich in them to make a regular part of what you eat.

Avocados are a wonderful source of monounsaturated fats (80 percent), as well as protein (10–15 percent), and range of micronutrients. But they have no starch and very little sugar (just 2 percent). Avocados contain fourteen minerals, including iron and copper, which help in red blood cell regeneration. They are nutrient-dense, containing more of a variety of nutrients than many other vegetables and fruits. Avocados have more potassium than bananas, without all the sugar. They are rich sources of the phytochemicals phytosterol, which inhibits cholesterol absorption and so lowers cholesterol levels, and glutathione, which has antacid properties. Avocados are also one of the richest sources of lutein, which protects against cancer and eye diseases. UCLA research shows that avocados have twice as much vitamin E as previously thought, making them the highest fruit source of that powerful acid buffer. I recommend eating at least one a day (more is certainly OK—and up to three to five is recommended if you have serious health conditions).

Coconuts, particularly young green coconuts and coconut water, are another excellent source of good saturated fats. Coconuts are 70 percent fat, and 90 percent of that fat is saturated, while the other 10 percent is monounsaturated. Those saturated fats have given coconut a bad rap recently. But the truth is, whole natural coconut and cold-pressed coconut oils are good for you. It is only when coconut is heated, processed, and hydrogenated that the saturated fats turn into trans fat, which *is* harmful. (So steam-fry your food first, and add your oils, including coconut oil, off the heat.) The good fats in whole natural coconut actually help *lower* cholesterol and *prevent* arteriosclerosis, rather than increase them, as the allegations went. Coconut is 15 percent protein, and is a complete protein.

Research shows that eating coconut does not lead to high cholesterol, increased heart disease, or increased mortality. Islanders with high intake of coconut oil showed no harmful effects, but when groups migrated to New Zealand and had less coconut oil in their diet, their total and bad cholesterol levels went up while their good cholesterol levels fell. When unsweetened coconut milk or coconut oil is added to an otherwise standard American diet, many studies show there is no change in cholesterol levels—while others show a drop. Rats fed a diet rich in safflower oil had six times higher cholesterol than did animals fed coconut oil instead.

Coconut milk, made by liquefying the white meat of the fruit, is very close to human breast milk in pH and fat and nutrient content. It is an excellent source of phosphorus, calcium, and iron. It provides a natural sweetness without much sugar. You have to take care to get natural, unsweetened coconut milk that isn't full of additives and preservatives.

Coconut water, extracted right from the hollow in the center of the nut, measures the same pH as human blood and is similar in molecular structure. It was actually used during World War II in place of blood plasma for transfusions when blood wasn't available.

Incorporate coconut water or milk into your salad dressings, and see the recipes chapter for many other ideas on how to use coconut. When choosing coconut oil, be sure to get one that is cold-pressed.

Fresh fish is rich in omega-3s as well as protein and many micronutrients. Like all animal protein, it contains no fiber and forms acid in your body when digested, so you can't eat it every day. But the benefits of the good fats it contains make this an important food to include in your diet. You must make sure it is absolutely fresh: newly caught, and with no "fishy" smell. And it must come from unpolluted waters. Salmon, trout, tuna, striped bass, and red snapper are among your best choices.

Seed oils like flax, borage, hemp, and primrose are high in good polyunsaturated fats. Make sure to get cold-pressed oils, as heat destroys nutrients.

Green Vegetables

Vegetables provide the vast majority of your body's needs: vitamins, minerals, fiber, and even macronutrients like protein and fats. Some of their lesser-known components are just as critical for good health:

- *Chlorophyll*, which gives green plants their green color, helps the blood deliver oxygen throughout the body. I call it the blood of plants because chlorophyll is very similar to human blood in both chemical components and molecular structure, with just one central atom differing between a molecule of each. Leafy greens are especially high in chlorophyll.
- *Metabolic co-factors* are what your body uses for every chemical activity in the body. There are thousands of co-factors, each with its own properties and functions, and eating a variety of vegetables provides your body with a variety of them. Co-factors also aid in digestion. Heat alters these co-factors, which is why having as many of your vegetables as possible raw is important. When you do cook your veggies, the less you do so, the better.
- *Phytonutrients* give some plants their yellow, orange, and red colors. They help neutralize acids, act as antioxidants, and help chromium bind to sugar for energy, along with other "co-factor" roles.

You can't go wrong choosing green vegetables like cucumber, celery, greens, the ones detailed here, and the many included on the exhaustive listing near the end of the chapter. To give you just a couple examples of the benefits that await you:

Broccoli is a great source of vitamin C; 14 ounces give just about all of the recommended daily allowance. It also contains folate, vitamin A, iron, potassium, vitamin B_6, magnesium, and riboflavin, all of which your body needs. Broccoli is an excellent source of fiber, and it helps balance blood sugar levels, lower cholesterol, improve digestion, strengthen the immune system, and control weight. Like all the green and yellow vegetables, broccoli has a pH between 7.5 and 8.

Spinach is at least as good for you as it is for Popeye. It is high in vitamin A, folate, iron, magnesium, calcium, vitamin C, riboflavin, potassium, and vitamin B_6. It is a great source of fiber and helps control blood sugar levels. Spinach also helps lower blood pressure and cholesterol, improve digestion, and increase immunity, and it assists in weight loss. In addition, spinach, too, has a pH between 7.5 and 8.

Choose fresh vegetables, always, and organic whenever you can. Eat them raw, preferably, and when you cook them, do it for as short a time as possible and at no higher than 118 degrees Fahrenheit if you can (enzymes survive up to that point).

Sprouts are not always green, but they are just about the best food you can eat. Filled with vitamins, minerals, and complete (and easily digestible) proteins, they are also high in enzymes, nucleic acids, and vitamin B_{12}, which is otherwise hard to find in vegetarian sources. Seeds become more alkaline as they sprout. And there is an explosion of nutrients as they sprout. Folic acid increases by 600 per-

EATING OUT

This plan goes with you wherever you go. You can get a salad pretty much anywhere these days, even in fast-food restaurants. In finer establishments, check out the appetizers for that 20 to 30 percent of your plate, and get a big salad besides. Ask for what you want; most restaurants will accommodate you, fixing a plate of steamed vegetables or leaving out an ingredient. To simplify things, use the little word "allergic" (as in, "I am allergic to mushrooms, please don't use any in the stir-fry").

If you're going to be flying, call ahead to request a pure vegan meal, and you will get something you can eat (and bring along a big bottle of green drink—flying is very dehydrating!).

In general, make it a habit to always have a little snack with you. This will help prevent you from becoming ravenously hungry and indulging in acidic foods, foods you would avoid if you weren't so hungry or had an alkaline alternative at the ready.

cent at sprouting, for instance, and riboflavin by about 1,300 percent! Move beyond the familiar alfalfa and bean sprouts to include in your diet sprouted lentils, broccoli, chickpea, sesame seeds, sunflower seeds, buckwheat, wheat, soy, and more. Try sprouting your own—just about any bean, grain, or seed.

Other Alkaline Foods

There are tons of alkaline foods you can choose from, as you'll see when you get to the long listing of them closer to the end of this chapter, but here I'd like to describe just a few of the truly great ones (in terms of benefits, but also in terms of utility).

Lemons, limes, and **grapefruit** are very low in sugar (3 percent, 3 percent, and 5 percent, respectively). Although they are chemically acid, they have an alkalizing effect when metabolized in the body. Squeeze some into your water throughout the day to help maintain your body's delicate pH balance.

Tomatoes also have very little sugar (3 percent) and, when eaten raw, are very alkalizing. Cooked, however, they become mildly acid-forming upon metabolism. They are rich in vitamins, as well as a substance called lycopene, which is the stuff that makes tomatoes red. It isn't made in the human body, though the body needs it. Lycopene has gotten a lot of attention for protecting against prostate cancer. It is also an acid buffer.

Good grains are steamed and sprouted—and whole. Quinoa, and raw buckwheat, to take just two examples, are high in protein and are excellent choices to round out a meal of green veggies and good fats.

Salt. It may surprise you almost as much to find salt recommended in this plan as it does to find fat. But sodium in its crystalline structure is a foundational element that keeps you alkaline. Your cells need to be bathed in saltwater. Healthy blood is salty—nearly as salty as the ocean—and the alkaline salts therein are used to neutralize acids in the blood. Salt is important to keeping your metabolism high. Metabolism is the production of energy when electron-rich alkaline water transfers from one cell to another—a process that is managed by the salt concentration in the cells. Water always moves from a cell with a lower salt concentration (energy potential) to a cell with a higher salt concentration (energy potential) as the body seeks pH balance.

You probably blame water retention for some of your excess weight and, in turn, blame the water retention on too much salt. But your body *retains* water because it is dehydrated, to dilute acids. When you are retaining water, it is a signal that your sodium is being converted into potassium in the body to balance your pH, and you actually need *more* water, and alkaline salts, like sea salt (e.g., Celtic Salt, or RealSalt from the Great Salt Lake). The problem is, Americans in general get way too much salt in their diets—the wrong kinds of salts. We salt just about everything we prepare, then keep salt on the table to add even more. Just about all prepared and processed foods are extremely salty. Table salt, and the salt added to just about all processed foods, has itself been overly processed, destroying its electrical potential. It has no electron energy. So while you do actually need to cut out all regular added salt from your diet, you then need *good* salt, electron-rich alkaline crystalline salt, like RealSalt or Celtic Salt. I recommend at least 3 to 4 grams a day.

Pamela

I have been overweight for most of my life. I've tried dozens of diets, lost weight—and put it right back on. Then the past few years, I just could not get the weight off no matter what I did. I weighed 337 pounds, had joint pain, and was always tired. At age fifty-seven, I knew it was just a matter of time before something really major happened. I have three beautiful grandchildren whom I want to see grow up.

So when I heard about going alkaline to lose weight, I decided to give it a try. I lost 10 pounds in the first eight days, just by eating 80 percent raw vegetables. It was at that point that I chose to really change my lifestyle. After just one month drinking green drink with pH drops, I had more clarity and less joint pain, and my energy level had greatly improved. I had lost 55 pounds by the end of twelve weeks. Now, after twenty-two months, I have lost 152 pounds! I have noticed other benefits: My hair is getting darker and showing a natural curl, for example. I've been able to buy new clothes since I no longer try to hide my fat, and I now can wear a size 14 dress, having gone from a size 2X top to a size small.

Using Shelley Young's recipes, I have been giving "uncooking" classes showing people how good eating raw food can be. My nine-year-old granddaughter will ask me if the food she is eating is healthy. I try to guide her in making food choices. And now I know I'll be around to see that payoff as she grows!

Acidic Foods

Foods that are themselves acidic, or have acidic effects on the body once they are digested, are better avoided if you wish to reach your ideal weight—and stay there. Be aware of the following acidic foods.

Animal Protein

Consumption of animal foods, including meat and dairy, has been linked to increased risk of heart disease (and increased risk of dying of heart disease) and cancer. (Vegetable-based diets examined in the same study showed no such increased risks.)

In addition: Eating **meat** stimulates insulin release—an even bigger release than pasta or popcorn—so you can't escape the dangers of blood sugar fluctuations by simply avoiding carbohydrates. Humans cannot fully digest meat, and as it goes through your system partially digested it damages the intestinal villus, leading to poor blood production and then poor body cell production.

There are many reasons for avoiding animal foods, not least of which is that it is simply *dead*. Anatomically and physiologically, humans are just not carnivores or omnivores; we are designed for the slow absorption of complex and stable plant food. That's why we have long and complicated digestive tracts, rather than the short, simple bowels of meat eaters, designed for minimum transit time. We have intestinal flora different from that of true carnivores. We don't have the teeth and jaws meant for tearing apart flesh.

It is yeast that causes the aging of meat, to get the final desired taste and texture. All meats "properly" aged for human consumption are partially fermented, and as such are permeated with acids and acid-generating microforms. Especially in the United States, animals are super-fattened with hormones, and the residues and acids from such accumulate in the fat. Red meat intake has been associated with increased risk of colon cancer, and consumption of animal fat has been linked to prostate, breast, and other cancers.

Pork is loaded with acid; pigs have no lymphatic system to move them out of the body, so metabolic acids are just stored in their tissues—your meat.

Like almost all meat grown in the United States, pork will have high levels of contamination by bacteria, yeast, and fungi and associated waste products and acids. For one thing, the grain these animals are fed is stored long term in silos, which are characteristically contaminated with fungi. Slaughterhouse conditions are also generally not sufficiently sanitary to protect against further contamination. Studies show that the majority of mycotoxins in meat are heat tolerant, so cooking won't protect you from them.

It should go without saying, but you must also try to avoid all processed, pickled, and smoked meats such as sausage, hot dogs, corned beef, luncheon meats, ham, bacon, pastrami, and pickled tongue or feet.

Chicken, according to Consumers Union, the advocacy group behind *Consumer Reports,* runs about a 42 percent chance of contamination by *Campylobacter jejuni,* and 12 percent of contamination by *Salmonella enterides,* numbers which USDA research confirms. Should you need another reason not to eat large quantities of chicken or turkey, consider that they do not urinate, which means they absorb their own acidic urine into their fleshy tissue instead. Large intakes of poultry have been associated with an increased risk of colon cancer.

One **egg** contains over 37,500,000 pathological microforms. You can see the effects of one egg in the blood—increased bacteria and yeast—within fifteen minutes of eating it, and it can take white blood cells up to seventy-two hours to clean up the mess. Eggs from grain-fed chickens have been documented to contain acids. Eating eggs at the rate of at least one a day has been associated with an increased risk of colon cancer.

Dairy products, including milk, cheese, ice cream, cottage cheese, and yogurt, have concentrated sugars called lactose. This lactose breaks down in the body to lactic acid, which causes irritation and inflammation in the muscles, bones, and joints. A high intake of dairy products, especially cheese and milk, has been associated with increased risk of breast and colon cancer.

HOW WILL I BUILD MUSCLE WITHOUT LOTS OF PROTEIN?

I know a lot of you are going to be thinking "But eating like this, where am I going to get my protein?" Your true concern should be if you, like almost all Americans, eat way too much protein. The average American man eats 175 percent more protein than the recommended daily allowance, whereas the average American woman goes over by 144 percent. That's from the 1988 Surgeon General's Report on Nutrition and Health—meaning we were already overdosing by that much *before* the high-protein diet craze hit. All the aminos you need for your body to make complete proteins are found in plant sources.

Furthermore, you don't need protein to build muscle. You need healthy blood to build muscle. And you build healthy blood with electron-rich green food and good fats, not protein. The strongest animals in the world—horses, gorillas, elephants—are plant eaters. And they sure aren't eating steak or having protein shakes for breakfast!

WHAT WILL HAPPEN TO MY BONES
IF I DON'T EAT DAIRY?

I think I get this question just about every day. But the truth is, the United States, England, and Sweden have the highest rates of osteoporosis in the world—and the highest level of milk consumption. American women have been getting an average of 2 pounds of milk per day for their entire lives (counting the milk that is concentrated in the process of making cheese, ice cream, yogurt, and milk), yet thirty million of them have osteoporosis. Drinking milk does not prevent bone loss. That's because bone loss is caused by too much protein intake. In 1986, *Science* magazine called dietary protein the most important contributor to osteoporosis. *The American Journal of Clinical Nutrition* in 1995 explained that "dietary protein increases production of acid in the blood which can be neutralized by calcium mobilized from the skeleton." A study in the *Journal of Nutrition* in 1981 found that doubling your protein intake doubled your calcium loss. And a 1979 study in the *American Journal of Clinical Nutrition* found that even someone getting 1,400 mg of calcium daily can lose up to 4 percent of their bone mass each year on a high-protein diet. The key is not to keep drinking milk for the calcium (getting more and more protein all the while) but to reduce the excess protein in your diet so that the body has no need to leach calcium from the bones to neutralize metabolic acids, weakening them.

Sweeteners

Sugar is a major contributor to acid production in the body, and a major contributor to obesity. And Americans eat fifty million pounds of the stuff every week.

When you eat sugar, the extra that isn't used for energy is fermented into acids, such as acetylaldehyde, a neurotoxin and lactic acid that, if not eliminated, can cause cell breakdown, and into ethanol alcohol in the liver, which also contributes to cellular breakdown. In contrast, my research shows that a diet low in sugar will result in a body low in acid.

You have to watch out for plain old white sugar, of course, as well as all the other forms of sugar: honey, maple syrup, brown sugar, molasses, corn syrup, and more. All the simple carbohydrates are handled in the body just like sugar, so you also need to eliminate white flour, white rice, pasta, and so on. These can all, like sugar, cause an overly rapid rise in blood sugar. Always check labels for sugars; they are in the majority of packaged foods, even ones you might not suspect. Another good reason to make whatever you eat yourself!

Artificial sweeteners like aspartame (NutraSweet), saccharin (Sweet'n Low), and sucralose (Splenda), break down into potentially deadly acids in the body. For example, when you ingest aspartame, one of the ingredients, methyl alcohol, converts into formaldehyde, a neurotoxin and known carcinogen! But that's not all. From there, it turns into formic acid, the same stuff fire ants use in their attacks. And that's just accounting for one ingredient in just one of the artificial sweeteners.

Aspartame is particularly bad when it comes specifically to contributing to obesity. The acid component the sweetener is named after (aspartic acid) is structurally and functionally quite close to that of the glutamic acid found in monosodium glutamate (MSG)—which in turn can contribute to weight gain.

If you must have a sweetener, safer options are the herbs stevia and chicory, available at natural food stores.

Peanuts

Peanuts are highly acidic and contain over twenty-seven yeasts and molds. When I first wrote this, I listed all twenty-seven, and it took the next six lines of text to do so. Don't eat them! (And that includes peanut butter.)

Corn

Corn contains twenty-five different fungi, including recognized carcinogens.

Yeast

You need to avoid both brewer's and baker's yeast, as well as "nutritional" yeast, along with all yeast-containing foods, like beer, wine, and bread and other baked goods. Eating yeast in any form can spur microform overgrowth in your body and increase their toxic acidic wastes. Read labels carefully to make sure all your foods, condiments, and seasonings are yeast-free.

Fermented and Malted Foods

This includes soy sauce, vinegar, miso, mayo, tamari, tempeh, olives, and pickles, as well as common condiments with one or more of those ingredients, like mustard, ketchup, steak sauce, prepared salad dressings, relish, and chili sauce. All are acidic, or acidic in the body, and fermented by fungus. Soy sauce, for example, has a pH of 4.45. You also need to eliminate malted products, which are also fermented by fungus (and contain a high level of sugar) and are acidic.

Alcohol

Alcohol is fermented and acidic. It will make you fat. Just think of the "beer belly"—and the fact that beer (even "lite" or "low-carb" beer) has a pH of about 4.5. Wine coolers are even worse; besides all the sweeteners, you're looking at a pH of 2.84.

All alcohol is a waste product made by bacteria or yeast. On top of that, the liver can convert alcohol into yet another toxic waste product—the acid acetylaldehyde.

The damage abuse of alcohol can do is already well known, of course, but the acid it contains does harm at even low levels.

Caffeine

One milligram of caffeine, injected directly into the bloodstream, can kill you. So there's enough in 1 ounce of milk chocolate to do in six people, and enough in a cup of strong coffee to off two hundred more. That ought to give you enough second thoughts to eliminate this addictive poison from your diet, but I also want to point out that caffeine is dehydrating. You need to be fully hydrated to reach and maintain your ideal weight, and you'll never get hydrated if you keep on using caffeine.

CAFFEINE CONTENT

Milk chocolate (1 oz.)	6 milligrams (mg)
Cola (12 oz. can)	36 mg
Anacin (2 tablets)	64 mg
Jolt (12 oz. can)	71.5 mg
Tea (8 oz. cup—weak)	20 mg
Tea (8 oz. cup—strong)	110 mg
Coffee (8 oz. cup—weak)	65 mg
Coffee (8 oz. cup—strong)	200 mg
Vivarin (1 tablet)	200 mg

Coffee

Even when you don't count the caffeine, coffee is no good for you. Coffee with cream and sugar has a pH of 4.0—1,000 times as acidic as distilled water. Black is a little better at 5.09, and decaf is slightly better still at 5.22. But acid is acid, and at those levels none of it belongs in a healthy body. If you're still not convinced, consider this: Research has shown that cancer cells can live indefinitely in coffee!

Tea

Once again, even if you're drinking "decaf" (which, like coffee, still contains some caffeine), the acidity of the beverage should take it off your menu: regular black tea comes in at 2.79, and green tea at 4.6.

Soft Drinks

First, most soft drinks are full of sugar and other sweeteners, and that right there should be enough for you to stop drinking them. And if they aren't full of sugar and corn syrup, then they are full of artificial sweeteners, which you should also avoid. Second, many soft drinks are caffeinated, another reason to skip them. Even those without caffeine are still bad, however, because of the acidity. Soda is saturated with protons, with a pH of about 3.0—10,000 times more acidic than distilled water. Sports drinks are among the worst—more acidic even than beer, as most sodas are. Gatorade Lemon/Lime for instance, has a pH of 2.95. Even soda water or seltzer with no sugar or artificial sweeteners or caffeine still contains carbonic acid, and has a pH of about 2.5—50,000 times more acidic than distilled water.

One of the key components of cola is phosphoric acid, which has a pH of 2.5. That's strong enough to dissolve a nail in about four days. To carry concentrated cola syrup, truckers must use the Hazardous Material designation reserved for highly corrosive materials. In your body, phosphoric acid leaches calcium from your bones, making it a major contributor to the rising increase in osteoporosis.

Americans guzzle an average of 44 gallons of soft drinks each year—an increase of 131 percent since the late 1970s. Forty-six percent of children aged six to eleven now drink soda every single day. No wonder we are so fat! We are pouring acid down our throats at quite a clip.

That's bad enough as it is, but remember that the more we drink of sodas, the less we drink of what is good for us. The National Soft Drink Association noted that Americans bought and drank four times as much soda as water.

Even if that ratio were flipped, we'd still be in trouble. Since it takes 20 parts bicarbonate to neutralize 1 part carbonic acid (which is in sodas), you'd have to drink 20 cups of alkaline water to counter just 1 cup of soda, diet or not, caffeinated or not. And more water on top of that to deal with acids from all other sources!

Product	pH
Sunny Delight	2.81
Gatorade	2.95
Coca-Cola	2.51
Diet Coke	2.97
Vanilla Diet Coke	2.95
Red Bull Energy	3.26
Twin Lab Ultra	2.83
Ripped Force	3.22
Snapple	2.83
Power Bars	2.93
7-Up	3.25

HYDRATE WITH ALKALINE WATER ONLY

You must supply your body with the hydration it needs only with alkaline water. Do not fall for proposed substitutes like sports drinks, which are all acidic and will only create the need for even more water in the body. Being overweight is a hallmark of being dehydrated or of trying to hydrate with acidic fluids. On the flip side, hydrating with good alkaline water is the first and most important step to reaching your ideal weight!

Chocolate

It's got sugar. It's got caffeine. It's got theobromine and methyl bromine, two very toxic acids. It makes you fat. You don't need it.

Fruit

Most fruits are high in sugar, and so, despite the nutrients they also contain, are best avoided. Pineapples are 28 percent sugar; bananas, 25 percent; honeydew melons, 21 percent; apples, 15 percent; oranges, 12 percent; strawberries, 11 percent; and watermelons, 9 percent—just to give you a few examples. That much sugar will keep your body acidic. You will not lose weight, or lose it quickly, or keep it off, if you are eating high sugar fruits. (As you'll see in the upcoming full listing of foods, some fruits are better than others, and you'll find a few I recommend there and in the previous section on alkaline foods.)

My research shows that one 8-ounce glass of fresh orange juice has enough sugar to create an acidic internal environment in the body and shut down up to half of white blood cell activity, reducing immune system function, for three to five hours. Apple juice, too, was acidic and toxic to the blood cells because of high sugar content. I've found that when I take my clients off high sugar fruits their red blood cells no longer stick together, causing circulation problems, and their white blood cells are more active and healthier. The clients begin to lose weight because they are reducing the acidity of their blood.

Mushrooms

Mushrooms of all kinds—shiitake, portobello, white, wild—must be avoided. For one thing, they are fungi. For another, they are acidic as they are digested.

Monosodium Glutamate

Glutamic acid in MSG is, first of all, an acid. Animal studies show it can cause brain lesions and neuroendocrine disorders, leading, in animals that ingest it, to gross obesity. A recent search of the Medline database through the National Library of Medicine using the key words "obesity AND monosodium glutamate" returned 143 references, with titles like "Obesity induced by monosodium glutamate in mice" (from *National Institute of Animal Health Quarterly*), "Brain lesions, obesity, and other disturbances in mice treated with monosodium glutamate" (from *Science*), and "The induction of obesity in rodents by means of monosodium glutamate" (from the *British Journal of Nutrition*). That's right: When scientists want to study obesity, one popular technique is to use MSG to fatten up the mice they are working with. As the title of one article specified, one injection of MSG is enough to wreak havoc on an animal.

There's no real reason the human animal should be any different. And the proportion of processed and packaged foods containing MSG is staggering. Fast foods, low- and no-fat foods, canned foods, and frozen foods are all likely to harbor glutamic acid. Eating the typical American diet, you are guaranteed to be dosing yourself with MSG and glutamic acid. If you want to shed your fat, you're going to have to get rid of this one "secret ingredient" that's helping to make and keep you fat.

CHOOSE YOUR FOODS

The following chart divides commonly eaten foods into six categories ranging from highly alkaline to highly acidic. For successful healthy weight loss, choose your foods mainly from those that are mildly to highly alkaline; do so and you will begin losing weight and other symptoms associated with excess acidity immediately. Avoid the acidic foods. Cut anything highly acidic out of your diet altogether, and keep foods in the mildly to moderately acidic categories to no more than 20 percent of your diet. If you want to be sure to lose weight and lose it fast, while remaining healthy, do not cross the line into the acidic foods.

ALKALINE—Electron-rich			ACID—Proton-rich			
	Best	Better	Good	Bad	Worse	Worst
	Highly Alkaline	Moderately Alkaline	Mildly Alkaline	Mildly Acidic	Moderately Acidic	Highly Acidic
Beans and legumes (non-stored)	soy nuts soy lecithin	lima beans soybeans (edamame) white navy beans granulated soy (cooked, ground soy-beans)	lentils soy flour tofu	seitan chickpeas kidney beans black beans		
Beverages	alkaline water		distilled water		fruit juice, natural	alcohol liquor fruit juice, sweetened beer tea coffee wine
Condiments	RealSalt Celtic Salt	red pepper cayenne garlic ginger onion	herbs most spices	curry powder	ketchup nutmeg vanilla table salt mayonnaise	mustard vinegar rice syrup soy sauce MSG jam jelly yeast malt cocoa carob
Fats (choose cold pressed)			olive oil borage oil coconut oil avocado oil flaxseed oil evening primrose oil marine lipids cod liver oil	sunflower oil grapeseed oil canola oil	margarine butter ghee corn oil	

	Best	Better	Good	Bad	Worse	Worst
	Highly Alkaline	Moderately Alkaline	Mildly Alkaline	Mildly Acidic	Moderately Acidic	Highly Acidic
Fruit			lime	plum	orange	dried fruit
			lemon	fresh date	banana	pickled fruit
			grapefruit	sweet cherry	pineapple	
			coconut	currant	peach	
			sour cherry	nectarine	watermelon	
				cantaloupe	honeydew	
					mango	
					apple	
					blackberry	
					fresh fig	
					dewberry	
					longberry	
					persimmon	
					guava	
					cherimoya	
					apricot	
					papaya	
					mango	
					tangerine	
					currant	
					gooseberry	
					grape	
					cranberry	
					strawberry	
					blueberry	
					raspberry	
Grains, non-stored			quinoa	millet	brown rice	barley
			buckwheat	kasha	wheat	corn
			groats	triticale	wild rice	rye
			spelt	amaranth	white rice	oat bran
					oats	
					white bread	
					biscuit	
					whole-meal bread	
					whole-grain bread	
					rye bread	

	Best	Better	Good	Bad	Worse	Worst
	Highly Alkaline	Moderately Alkaline	Mildly Alkaline	Mildly Acidic	Moderately Acidic	Highly Acidic
Meat, poultry, and fish				freshwater fish, wild (not farm raised)	ocean fish, wild (not farm raised)	shellfish farm-raised fish pork veal beef chicken poultry eggs organ meats
Milk and milk products	human breast milk		goat milk	soymilk rice milk milk cream		hard cheese cottage cheese ice cream yogurt soy cheese goat cheese whey casein (milk protein)
Nuts			almond	brazil nuts hazelnuts pecans	walnuts	pistachios peanuts cashews
Root vegetables		beets radish ginger	rutabaga horseradish turnip carrot			potatoes (stored)
Seeds	pumpkin		sesame cumin fennel caraway	sunflower flax		
Sweeteners			stevia chicory			artificial sweeteners saccharin aspartame white sugar beet sugar corn syrup molasses

	Best	Better	Good	Bad	Worse	Worst
	Highly Alkaline	Moderately Alkaline	Mildly Alkaline	Mildly Acidic	Moderately Acidic	Highly Acidic
						dried sugar cane
						cane juice
						barley malt syrup
						fructose
						turbinado sugar
						brown rice syrup
						maple syrup
						honey
Vegetables	grasses	tomato	brussels sprouts			mushroom
	sprouts	avocado	peas			
	dandelion	green beans	asparagus			
	soy sprouts	sorrel	artichokes			
	cucumber	spinach	comfrey			
	sea vegetables	garlic	cauliflower			
	broccoflower	celery	zucchini			
	kale	cabbage	rhubarb			
	parsley	lettuce	leeks			
		bell peppers	watercress			
		collard greens	chives			
		broccoli	kohlrabi			
		endive				
		arugula				
		mustard greens				
		okra				

PUTTING IT TOGETHER

With all that in mind, exactly how are you going to fill your plate? The key is to make the foundation of every meal electron-rich green foods and mono- and polyunsaturated fats. These are the foods that will build healthy blood and maintain the alkalinity of your body. Cover 60 to 80 percent of your plate with them, with smaller amounts of grains, beans, soy, fish, and cooked vegetables. Our bodies are designed to operate on fuel in this proportion, about 80 percent of it alkaline.

So think of your ideal meal as basically a big salad, with cooked or less alkaline foods "on the side." But don't think of that salad as a boring pile of iceberg lettuce and tomato. With the recipes in this book to guide you, you'll soon discover the almost infinite variety available to the creative salad maker. Using a range of colors, textures, and flavors, you'll enjoy delicious and satisfying meals on this plan. Dressings alone can take you to every country in the world and

---

Mark

For years now I've felt terribly addicted to sweets and candy. I've tried many different diet plans to try to get rid of the extra weight I was carrying. More recently I started getting bad heartburn often. I then tried "hot yoga," which actually helped a lot with the heartburn. But I actually began to gain weight! I was still craving sugar and thought I could afford to indulge because of the yoga.

Fortunately I found the pH Miracle plan. This is the one program that really makes sense to me. I've shed the 13 pounds I needed to lose. And I feel so much more alive.

I'm excited about preparing food now. I've never really cooked or been that interested in it before. But in just the past week I've made hummus and salsa and even some more adventurous dishes. I love the look of the salads I'm making. Such great colors!

I did a weeklong "cleanse," and during that time took three 90-minute yoga classes. The combination was amazing! By the third class, on the fifth day of the cleanse, the improvement in my yoga was remarkable. I was getting into poses that a week before had seemed impossible for me to achieve. I can hardly believe it myself that a change of diet would make me more flexible, but that is exactly what's happened.

back again; because of the healthy oils they contain, and the concentrated seasonings and flavor, you should consider them a major part of your meal. Experiment with different herbs and spices. Use the recipes in this book as a springboard to your own creations, mixing and matching, substituting one ingredient for another, adding or deleting items as you go. Pay attention to how you arranged your salad. We enjoy our food with all our senses, not just taste, and presentation is part of what makes any given meal so appealing.

As your taste buds and your system become accustomed to this way of eating, you will lose your appetite for acidic foods. The more acidic you are, the more acidic foods you will crave. But the more alkaline you eat, the more alkaline your body will be, the more energy you will have—and the more your body will crave more of that energy and that alkaline food. The better you feel, the better you'll understand how the acidic foods pull you down, making you tired and sick, and you simply won't want them anymore. You won't want to feel the way they make you feel. And the energy eating this way brings you will make you more active, the other key pillar in any weight-loss plan. Finally, as you will be providing your body with all that it needs, and exactly what it needs, it will require less food intake in general, and you'll naturally eat less without doing so consciously and without ever feeling unsatisfied.

As you practice the alkalizing principles in this book, you will watch the numbers on the scale go down to where you want them to be—and stay there. Moreover, you'll have more energy and vibrant health than you've ever experienced before. You'll look better, too, and not only because of the weight dropping off: The glow of good health will shine through. Good eating habits are essential not just to staying alive, but also to living.

Chapter 9

Basic Supplements

For me, a landscape does not exist in its own right, since its appearance changes at every moment; but the surrounding atmosphere brings it to life, the air and the light, which vary continually . . . for me, it is only the surrounding atmosphere that gives subjects their true value.
—CLAUDE MONET

Even with a very good diet, supplements are an important weight-loss tool. To some degree, supplements are like an insurance policy against nutrient deficiencies. Your diet may not be as good as you think it is. The nutritional quality of food has dropped considerably in the past few decades, as soils are depleted and lacking in vitamins, minerals, and trace nutrients. Many, many foods are processed in ways that rob them of more of their remaining nutritional value. Foods that are then cooked lose still more nutrients. The only way to be sure you are getting all the vitamins, minerals, and micronutrients you need is with supplements. This chapter details how to support healthy, natural—and permanent—weight loss with a basic (pun intended!) program of nine daily supplements that ensure you provide your body with all the nutrition it needs to keep itself healthy, alkaline, and lean. Of course, as with exercise or diet changes, before beginning any new supplements you should consult with your health care provider.

DRINK YOUR GREENS

Eating your veggies is a step in the right direction, but drinking them is even better. Stirring some **"green powder"** into good water will help you maintain a highly alkaline body like nothing else. Green powder is highly concentrated nutrition, and you get the benefits of pounds of vegetables, herbs, leaves, and grasses in every teaspoonful. Green powder is rich in electrons. (You can witness that if you use a plastic scoop to get it out of the bottle—the negatively charged green powder will cling to the positively charged plastic, the way opposites do.) So it is a powerful neutralizer of acids.

Green powder can provide over 125 easily absorbed vitamins and minerals, along with macronutrients including amino acids (protein) and fiber. (Green powder contains both soluble and insoluble fiber, though getting enough fiber is one thing you can count on from having your diet focused around green foods.) Another key ingredient

Steve

I am a thirty-six-year-old father of three, and up until I started drinking green drink, 212 pounds of flab. Then, in just two weeks, I lost 9 pounds. What was more impressive was the energy I gained, as well as the ability to sleep soundly. (If that wasn't enough, I actually stopped snoring!) I took this newfound energy with me to the gym and started working out. At the end of twelve weeks, I'd lost over 20 pounds of fat while picking up new muscle. I currently weigh 192 pounds and have the best body I've had since I played football in high school.

My wife has also been drinking her greens, and she looks amazing. She no longer smokes, drinks coffee, or has any caffeine, all things she has done for two decades. She has always been thin, but now her body is fit, firm, and healthy. She just glows.

green powder delivers is chlorophyll, the substance that makes plants look green and helps them absorb light. The molecular structure of chlorophyll is similar to that of hemoglobin, the substance in red blood cells that gives them their red color and helps them transport oxygen. They differ at the center of the atom, where hemoglobin has iron and chlorophyll has magnesium. Chlorophyll helps your blood deliver oxygen throughout the body, making stronger blood and thus stronger body cells.

Green powders vary in the specific types and amounts and ratios of nutrients they contain, depending on the ingredients included. The label on the product you are looking for might say "barley grass" or "kamut grass" in the biggest type, though you're looking for a blend of greens. You'll have plenty to choose among at your local natural food store. The following chart gives you an idea of the best ingredients to look for when choosing a green powder—you won't find all of them, but be sure to get a range of them. The one thing you must be sure your powder includes is a variety of grasses. All the good stuff you could say about green vegetables goes double for grasses, which are incredibly nutrient-dense. To give you just one example, wheat grass contains vitamins C, E, and K, as well as all of the B complex vitamins, one of the highest levels of vitamin A in any food, and every identified mineral and trace mineral. Not to mention that it is 25 percent protein!

You should also check with the manufacturer to make sure the green powder is made with-low heat dehydration, and not over-processed, so the electrons are not damaged or lost. And please make sure there are no algaes, mushrooms, yeasts, or probiotics (so-called healthy bacteria!) included; these are, unfortunately, common additions, but they are all acidifying.

Ingredients to Look for in Green Drinks

• alfalfa leaf	• golden seal leaf	• rosehips
• aloe	• kale leaf	• rosemary leaf
• avocado powder	• kamut grass	• sage
• barley grass	• lecithin	• shave grass
• beta carotene	• lemon grass	• slippery elm bark
• bilberry leaf	• marshmallow root	• spearmint leaf
• black walnut leaf	• meadowsweet	• spinach
• blueberry leaf	• oat grass	• strawberry leaf
• boldo leaf	• okra fruit	• thyme
• broccoli	• papaya leaf	• tomato leaf
• cabbage	• parsley	• turmeric
• celery	• pau d'arco root	• watercress
• couch grass	• peppermint leaf	• wheat grass
• dandelion leaf	• plaintain leaf	• white willow bark
• echinacea	• red raspberry leaf	• wintergreen leaf

pH RX

Stir 1 teaspoon of green powder into 1 liter of good alkaline water (see chapter 5), and drink at least 1 liter of the resulting "green drink" each day for every 30 pounds of body weight. You can add more greens if you like, especially if you are trying to build muscle.

Lisa

Over the course of seven years, I had sought the advice of at least twenty-eight medical professionals. I spent my life in the offices of M.D.'s, specialists, chiropractors, physical therapists, massage therapists, nutritionists, and acupuncturists.

Moreover, I spent $30,000 on treatments, therapies, and supplements in hopes of finding some relief from my chronic pain, allergies, and depression. I tried many different diets, including high protein/no sugar, complex carbs/no animal protein, vegetarian, vegan, and macrobiotic. Many approaches helped, but I was never free of physical and emotional pain.

Until I tried green drink. My body became more alkaline, and got rid of toxins in my body from stress and poor diet. Within one month, my pain was reduced by 85 percent. As a side benefit, I lost 15 pounds!

Eighteen months later, I've never felt better. I am free of pain, free of prescription medications (I'd been using three), free from blood sugar imbalances and mood swings, free of low energy and brain fog. Having gone from a size 12 to a size 4, I am also free from ever having to worry about fitting into my jeans!

GET FATS

When it comes to good fats (see chapter 6), once again what you get in your diet is crucially important, but probably not entirely sufficient for ideal results. Most Americans have low levels of omega-3 fatty acids. And their levels of omega-3s and omega-6s, which should be present in a pretty steady proportion to work well, are often out of whack, meaning either they are not getting the additional nutrients they need to metabolize the fats correctly, or they are not getting the fats in the right proportion in their diets (or both). Supplements of omega-3 and omega-6 fatty acids, used correctly, can restore and maintain that balance in the body. The good fats will help your body neutralize acids and eliminate them from the body, among the many benefits examined in chapter 6. They will also help curb your appetite. Fats trigger the sense of satiety, or fullness, without increasing acidity or draining your energy reserves.

Just as you have to choose the right fats, you need to choose the right fat supplements. To begin with, you must make sure you have fresh oil in the capsules. Just open the bottle and take a sniff. If it's rancid you'll smell it! Make sure your capsules contain adequate amounts of each of the three most significant omega-3 fats; ALA, EPA, and DHA: Those three should make up at least two-thirds of the product. The omega-6s LA, CLA, and GLA should make up a maximum of one-third (see chapter 6). And your supplement should provide the nutrient co-factors that ensure successful fat metabolism and properly balanced levels of stored fatty acids: a complete spectrum of antioxidants (another word for antacid), starting with vitamins C and E; vitamins B_3, B_6 and B_{12}, folic acid, and riboflavin; vitamins A and D; and the minerals magnesium and zinc. The manufacturer should be able to provide an independent analysis to verify the levels of all the nutritional components of their supplements.

Finally, your supplement needs to provide omega-6 and omega-3 essential fats in the proper ratio, which most experts consider to be 1:3—which is just the proportion in hemp oil. Most Americans have levels in their bodies of the stored essential fatty acids somewhere between 20 to 1 and 30 to 1. That's because omega-3s don't appear in many foods most Americans eat regularly, while omega-6s are plentiful in the typical diet. Following the pH Miracle plan,

TO FISH, OR NOT TO FISH, THAT IS THE QUESTION

I recommend getting your omega-3s from marine (fish) oils, which contain preformed omega-3s. You can get them from plant sources, but the body has to work to convert them. Especially if your system is weakened, that's a stress it could do without. In some cases, fish oils have been shown to have a stronger effect than the closest vegetarian equivalents (though in some cases, like addressing the symptoms of PMS, borage oil outperforms fish oils).

> **pH RX**
>
> Take 1 (1,000 mg) capsule with omega-6 and omega-3 fatty acids in a 1:3 ratio 6 to 9 times per day with alkaline water or green drink.
>   Take 1 (500 mg) capsule of CLA at least three times a day.

you'll be getting a balanced amount in your food, and doing so in your supplement is important as well.

I recommend getting ½ to 1 cup of good oil each and every day. That's very difficult to do, so I recommend using supplements.

SOY SPROUTS

Sprouted soybeans are filled with vitamins (including the "hard to find in vegetarian form" B_{12}), minerals, and enzymes. Soy sprouts are also an excellent plant source of protein. They are, in fact, 41 percent protein by volume—more than fish, pork, beef, chicken, or turkey. And the protein is complete—contains all the types of amino acids your body needs to build all its proteins—a rarity among plants.

Soy sprouts provide all the benefits of soy, including lowering cholesterol, inhibiting atherosclerosis, balancing sugar levels, and preventing osteoporosis and some types of cancer. But sprouts, unlike soybeans before sprouting, are alkaline and full of electrons. They also contain isoflavones, plant estrogens that help balance human hormones. It is the isoflavones that give soy its well-deserved reputation for alleviating menopausal and PMS symptoms. In balancing the endocrine system, preventing hormones from being overproduced, soy sprouts remove a form of food for bacteria and yeast to grow on.

In selecting a soy sprouts supplement, look for a low-heat dehydrated product.

Michael

I've suffered with a number of health conditions for twelve years. Being overweight is only one among more than a dozen complaints, ranging from arthritis and depression to reflux and allergies, the combination of which has rendered me so disabled that I haven't been able to work all that time.

All that changed when I started taking green drink with pH drops and powdered soy sprouts. I thought I had just about run out of options but decided on one last-ditch effort. I had tried many natural methods to relieve my symptoms, but nothing else ever worked effectively for the long term. I can say without any exaggeration that all of my conditions have disappeared, with 99 percent relief. It's a recovery I could only dream of just a year ago. I have abounding energy, my thinking has become much clearer, I can attend to details much more easily, and I am much less stressed. And I have lost 23 pounds!

pH RX

Take 1 teaspoon of soy sprout powder at least six times a day, or when you have sugar cravings.

pH DROPS

Truly good water (distilled or ionized, as detailed in chapter 5) can do wonders for your health, as you've seen, but if you want a real pH miracle you'll need to add in "pH drops"—sodium chlorite—or sodium bicarbonate (common baking soda) or sodium silicate. Stirring one of these into your water will not only raise the pH but also increase the level of oxygen and electrons. (See chapter 5 for the health benefits of the *right* water.)

You can buy sodium silicate or sodium chlorite at your natural food store. Choose pH drops that are clear, not cloudy, in the bottles. Cloudy pH drops have lost their potency.

---

pH RX

Add 2 to 3 teaspoons of sodium bicarbonate or 16 drops of 2 percent sodium chlorite to 1 liter of the right water. Ideally, you'd add it to all your water, along with the green powder.

Bruce

I am a registered nurse. I weighed 283 pounds and had a cholesterol level of 225 before beginning this program. My joints ached and I was tired all of the time. I was a mess!

When I first heard about the pH Miracle, I was skeptical of any diet program; I had tried high-protein diets and many others with no success. But I started using green drink, pH drops, soy sprouts, and Montmorillonite clay, and within five months I had lost 54 pounds. I went from size 42 pants down to size 36. My cholesterol dropped to 185. Just a year after I started, I am down to 225 and feeling great. My joints no longer ache and I feel more energized and focused. My coworkers have been astounded by my transformation. When they ask me about the "magic bullet" responsible, I always tell them this is a life-altering change that takes an inner strength to achieve.

L-CARNITINE

L-carnitine, which occurs naturally in the body, is invaluable because, pure and simple, it burns fat. Its job is to bind to fatty acids and transport them into your mitochondria—your cells' power stations—to be used as fuel. It's also a binder of metabolic acids. A deficiency will result in acids being stored in the fatty tissue and will make weight loss even more difficult. Low levels of L-carnitine may increase food intake. Conversely, taking L-carnitine promotes weight loss and lean muscle mass and decreases BMI and body fat content. It also decreases cravings and increases energy levels (making exercise easier).

One study looked at overweight patients over a twelve-week period. These patients ate a low-calorie diet and performed moderate exercise. Half the group was also given 2,000 mg of L-carnitine, while the others took a placebo. People taking the L-carnitine lost an average of 11 pounds, compared with just 1 pound in the placebo group. Body fat percentages also decreased markedly in the L-carnitine group. They also experienced lowered cholesterol, blood sugar levels, and blood pressure.

pH RX

Take 200 mg of L-carnitine six times a day.

GARCINIA CAMBOGIA/HCA

Hydroxic citric acid, or HCA, available as a standardized herbal extract of the fruit of the *Garcinia cambogia* plant, not only curbs your appetite, reducing the amount of food you eat, but also inhibits lypogenesis, the process by which the body produces and stores fat. It's especially good at reducing the increase of excess acids from the metabolism of complex carbohydrates and proteins in your diet, thus reducing the need for the body to store these acids in the body fat. The acids are bound up to the HCA and then eliminated through the urinary tract or the bowels. As a bonus: Because you are using those carbs and protein for energy and the acids created as a waste product from their metabolism are then bound up by HCA, you avoid the irritability, depression, and/or fatigue that can come with dramatic changes in blood sugar levels, and experience a more even supply of energy between meals. Researchers have used radioactive tracer studies to show that HCA cuts the body's fat storage ability by up to 75 percent. It also lowers the production of cholesterol and fatty acids. Animal studies show that HCA reduces the conversion of carbohydrates into stored acidic fat, suppresses appetite, and induces weight loss.

More than thirty years of studies in this country—and use from ancient times in India, where Garcinia cambogia is native—show virtually no side effects or evidence of toxicity of HCA on the body. Studies published over the years in a wide variety of scientific journals, including *Lipids, The American Journal of Clinical Nutrition, The American Journal of Physiology, Physiological Behavior,* and *The Journal of Biological Chemistry,* have shown, among other things, that using HCA significantly improved the results of dieting, even though the amount of food intake was not affected.

In addition, its appetite suppressant effects don't wear off, though the body develops tolerance to most such drugs in just a few days. HCA is as safe as it is effective, and will help the body, over time, reduce stored body fat—and increase energy levels.

This supplement might be labeled as Garcinia cambogia, or as HCA. There are only a few commercially available extracts of garcinia, and they vary in terms of quality. Look for an extract of Garcinia cambogia with standardized HCA content, preferably 50 percent by weight of pure hydroxic citric acid calcium salt. I recommend Citra-Max from the Health Corporation, which has the highest level of HCA; they import the Garcinia cambogia powder from India. Some other suppliers measure only total acidity of the extract without specifying the amount of HCA in particular.

Once you have a good source of HCA, be sure to take it a half an hour to an hour before eating a meal. You need to give your body time to absorb the HCA and put it to work. Studies show that tak-

---

pH RX

Take 3 (660 mg) capsules, with 50 percent by weight being HCA, thirty to sixty minutes before a meal, at least three times a day or before each meal.

---

ing it *with* a meal, or even two or three hours later, produces virtually no benefit.

CHROMIUM

The mineral chromium helps insulin metabolize fat, turn protein into muscle, and convert sugar into energy. It increases insulin's effectiveness, improving its ability to handle glucose (sugar), thereby regulating blood sugar levels. Chromium also reduces cravings for sugar and simple carbs, and it helps improve the muscle-to-fat ratio in the body's composition. All this contributes to easier weight control. Chromium has other benefits as well, notably influencing cholesterol levels, improving the condition of the arteries, and boosting energy levels by fighting fatigue.

Without enough chromium, your body can't burn off sugar properly, which will eventually result in hyperglycemia or hypoglycemia or diabetes. In the process, this remaining sugar will ferment to acid and store itself in the body fat, and you won't have enough energy. With your metabolism out of whack, and insulin production gone haywire, you'll gain weight more easily, among other problems.

Chromium becomes particularly important after age thirty-five. As we age, the human body tends to handle blood sugar less well, with cells having a harder time taking it up and burning it. At that point, chromium's assistance becomes absolutely crucial.

In a study published in *Nutrition Review* in 1998, 122 patients were given either 400 micrograms (mcg) of chromium picolinate per day, or a placebo. After ninety days, and after adjusting for caloric intake and expenditure, those who took chromium lost more weight (17.1 vs. 3.9 pounds), fat mass (16.9 vs. 3.3 pounds), and percentage of body fat (6.3 percent vs. 1.2 percent) than the placebo group. A trial at the Health and Medical Research Foundation also found that people taking chromium daily lost more body fat and gained more muscle mass over seventy-two days than did people in the study taking a placebo.

The National Academy of Science recommends a chromium intake of 50 to 200 mcg a day, but nine of ten American adults don't meet even the minimum level. A USDA survey in the late 1980s showed the average American man got about 33 mcg daily. He at least beat out the average woman, who got just 25 mcg a day—half the recommended minimum. The body doesn't do very well assimilating chromium from food—it gets just 1 to 2 percent of it. Our food tends to be lower in chromium than it used to be, and lower than it is in many other places in the world because our soil is depleted, so neither our water supply nor our crops get as much as desirable. Furthermore, refining food decreases its chromium content right along with the other nutrients it destroys. Overall, this deficiency is as rare in other countries as it is common in ours.

Meanwhile, studies show that helpful doses of chromium are more in the range of 200 to 800 mcg a day anyway. To reach that, Americans, at least, require supplements.

Look for a chromium supplement that is bound or coated with niacin rather than yeast, as in polynicotonate or amino acid–bound chromium picolinate. I have found that the most effective form of chromium is in the polynicotonate glucose tolerance factor (GTF).

pH RX

Take 200 mcg three times a day, ideally half yeast-free polynicotonate GTF and half chromium picolinate, which can generally be found together in one product. You can also take the colloidal or liquid form, 5 drops under the tongue six times a day.

TYROSINE

The amino acid tyrosine helps signal the brain to turn off the appetite, which helps you eat less. It is also a precursor for three major neurotransmitters, including adrenaline, and adrenal hormones, which are generally out of balance in an overweight person. Tyrosine influences normal or baseline metabolic rate, which helps in weight loss. Tyrosine helps reduce body fat.

I recommend the L-tyrosine form of tyrosine, as it is more bioavailable. You should take tyrosine on an empty stomach so that it won't be in competition for absorption and transportation to the brain with other amino acids you eat. As long as it gets a fair shot at it in this way, even a modest dose of tyrosine, taken regularly over time, can have a real effect.

Look for HCA formulated with chromium and L-tyrosine, or L-tyrosine formulated together with HCA and chromium; I'm all for reducing the number of pills you swallow by using combination supplements when appropriate.

---

pH RX

Take 500 mg one to two times a day. You can also take the liquid or colloidal form, 5 drops under the tongue six times a day.

CLAY

And now for something a bit more unusual: The final key in your natural weight loss plan is to eat dirt. Specifically, smectite Montmorillonite clay (it comes from Montmorillon, France). But before you turn up your nose at the idea, give me a minute to explain.

The right clay provides your body with an impressive assortment of alkaline minerals, including calcium, iron, magnesium, potassium, manganese, sodium, sulfur, and silica, in natural proportion to one another. It is highly negatively charged—full of electrons available to your body. Additionally, it can trap and absorb many times its weight in acids, holding them until your body can safely eliminate them—and keeping them from being stored in body fat. In fact, Montmorillonite clay, with its negative charge, attracts and absorbs many positively charged impurities in the body, like toxins and microforms, allowing the body to eliminate them, too, safely. Clay provides a range of benefits including improved digestion and elimination, better circulation, higher quality sleep, increased energy, decreased depression, and a stronger immune system. All of that on top of helping the body lose weight—and maintain a healthy weight.

Montmorillonite clay is the most common and the most sought after of the clays suitable for eating. It is available in most health food stores. Some clay will come formulated with other beneficial ingredients. I like the blend with aloe vera and grapeseed oil. Don't let the thought that you are eating clay put you off; clay has a neutral taste and, much like tofu, will take on the taste of what you eat it with.

pH RX

Take 1 teaspoon at least three times a day. You can take it as is, from the jar, or stir it into 4 to 6 ounces of water.

For optimal results, use all these supplements together. They support each other, buffering acids, acting as co-factors in a variety of biological functions, and providing building blocks for blood and then body cells. In short, they provide all the elements for maintaining an alkaline environment in the body, in and outside the cell—setting the stage for healthy, permanent weight loss.

Chapter 10

Let's Get Physical

*You will come to the grave in full vigor, like sheaves
gathered in season.*
—JOB 5:26

You can burn calories with any number of forms of exercise, but I'm
here to tell you you're not exercising in a way that's going to really
help you lose weight unless you are sweating. Sweating is one of
the major ways your body eliminates acids. Moving your body to the
point where you break a sweat promotes the pumping of the
lymphatic system, which serves to remove toxins and acidic wastes
from the tissues and fluids of the body and release them through the
skin. Sweating opens up your pores to allow acids in both liquid and
gas form to pass through. You've got 3,500 pores per square inch of
your skin. That's a lot of ways for acids to get out—if you give them
room. Toxins in gas form also leave the body through the lungs,
aided by increased rate of respiration with exercise.

If you don't do it properly, exercise can actually make your body
more acidic. That's right: Exercise could be making you fat. Unless
you know how to do it the right way. That's where this chapter comes
in. You'll learn how to exercise to remove excess acids through sweating and respiration, build healthy muscles, and ensure you're burning
the right kind of fuel to power all this efficiently and effectively. It

doesn't have to be any more complicated than walking, but you still need to understand the benefits of exercise—and how to achieve them—to make whatever exercise you choose work for you. The second half of this chapter provides the details of a specific program—The pH Miracle workout—ideal for alkalizing your body, keeping fit—and losing weight.

I don't have to tell you exercise is good for you. Or that you should consult your health care provider before beginning any exercise program. Getting and keeping your body in motion is famously good for your heart, and, of course, your muscles. It's good for your bones and your joints. Exercise helps prevent diabetes. It reduces stress and improves mood. In fact, exercise is crucial for good health and critical to reaching and maintaining a healthy weight. Exercise does burn calories, of course (even if that's not the main point: sweating is!). Moreover, it not only increases your metabolism while you are active, but also, by building muscle, speeds up even your resting metabolism. The key fact about exercise, often overlooked, is that it helps keep your body alkaline. But you have to do it right, or it will have the opposite effect.

BURN, BABY, BURN

One of the good things (even if it is not the *main* thing) about exercise is that it burns calories. The more you move, the more fuel your body burns. That fuel can come from your food—and it can come from the unwanted fat stored in your body. The more active you are, the more fuel you need. Providing your body with the correct amount of fuel (calories or, even better said, electrons) is one way to stay slim. Too many calories—and especially acidic calories (protons)—and your body will store rather than burn the excess fuel. The more fuel you burn (the more active you are) in relation to food you take in, the more stored fat will be burned off as fuel.

Muscles are the engines that burn the fuel. Exercise increases your muscle mass, and the more muscle mass you have, the higher your fuel requirement. The more muscle you have, the more fuel

> ## Amy
>
> I've been using green drink for a year now and am happy to report significant improvements in my health, my attitude toward my body, and my overall outlook on my life! My weight has always been just below average for my five-foot-nine frame, and with the greens and alkaline eating I lost body fat and gained muscle mass. My body fat dropped from 16 to 6 percent, but my weight didn't change. More important, I've begun to stop comparing my body to everyone else's. I am comparing the "old" me with the "new" me instead! And I am able to work out much more easily, and better. I've depended on a rescue inhaler for asthma since I was seven years old, and as an adult I have to interrupt a workout two or three times to use it. Now I don't need it at all! I'm also sleeping better. Finally, I've found a new dimension to my job as a mother, as a role model for healthy eating and hydrating.

you'll need and the more fuel you'll burn—whether you are in motion or at rest.

Burning the right fuel, as well as the right amount of fuel, is important to weight loss. Using fat, rather than sugar, as your main source of fuel—especially during exercise—will minimize acidity, thereby increasing energy, strength, and endurance. Burning fat produces six times the energy with half the acid compared to burning sugar or protein.

As your body burns its fuel—food—to release electron energy, carbon dioxide, which is actually a toxin (an acid), is created—and then expelled through the lungs. At least, that's what happens as long as you're getting plenty of oxygen. Without enough oxygen the mode of energy production shifts from respiration to fermentation, creating a much more toxic waste product, especially lactic acid.

Lactic acid can't just be breathed out; it is expelled into the surrounding tissues. When that happens, you experience pain, irritation, and/or inflammation.

It's this exact process that so many people *seek* when they exercise, believing in the "no pain, no gain" mantra so common in the fitness and body-building worlds. It's unfortunate so many people aim to get to the threshold of physical pain in order to build strength, size, and/or endurance. For one thing, this is a totally unnecessary experience of pain. Even more important, it's guaranteed to have exactly the opposite of the desired effect. Exercising in such a way as to make your body even more acidic will never make you lean, strong, and healthy.

Furthermore, it is important never to exercise to the point of exhaustion (that is, you feel exhausted and have soreness or pain in your muscles). Exhaustion from exercise can be systemic, or localized in a particular muscle or muscle group. When you feel that burning sensation in your muscles, you are over-exercising. Your muscles are exhausted, your body isn't getting enough oxygen, and you'll be getting more, rather than less, acidic as a result of your efforts. Signs that your exhaustion is getting more serious include tightness in the throat, reduced peripheral vision, light-headedness or dizziness, and, at the extreme, feeling faint, weak, or ready to pass out. Certain techniques or types of exercise—including long-distance running or swimming, excessive weight lifting, and spinning—can be very exhausting if not performed properly. Doing it right means never doing it to the point of exhaustion. Moreover, if you exercise to the point of pain, that's a key sign you are burning sugar rather than fat—and acidifying your body as you go.

Signs you are exhausted, over-exercising, and/or burning sugar as you exercise:

- Light-headedness
- Dizziness

- Cloudy thinking
- Cold hands or feet
- Tingling in the extremities
- Narrowing of peripheral vision
- Hearing yourself breathing
- Inhaling and exhaling through your mouth instead of your nose
- Feeling disconnected with your environment
- Burning sensations in your body
- Unable to carry on a conversation while exercising
- Your brow is furrowed and tight
- Your fists are clenched tightly
- Your muscles are tight
- You have a knot in your throat
- You become agitated or anxious
- Your sweat smells like ammonia
- Systemic or localized pain

Signs you are exercising correctly: moderately and aerobically, and burning fat while you exercise:

- Feeling peaceful
- Feeling grounded
- Feeling connected to your external environment
- Feeling no pain
- Feeling a sense of euphoria
- Clear thinking
- Able to carry on a conversation
- Facial expressions relaxed and happy

- Wide peripheral vision
- All senses are enhanced
- Inhaling and exhaling through your nose, not your mouth
- Breathing quietly and easily
- Feeling more flexible
- Feeling "in the zone"

The key to healthful exercise to provide an alkaline internal environment is to keep it aerobic, pain-free, and fat-burning. You can choose from a variety of light aerobic exercises, like walking, easy jogging, swimming, biking, or, my personal favorite as you'll see below, rebounding. Should you ever reach the point of pain, where you know you are burning sugar, you should stop immediately and drink a green drink or good alkaline water to restore alkalinity.

ON THE REBOUND

There's only one way I know of to guarantee that all 75 trillion cells in your body get the ideal workout all at once, and that's rebounding. Working out on a small, low trampoline applies weight and movement to every cell in the entire body, the most efficient way to become stronger, more flexible, healthier—and slimmer! Cells expand and contract with the vertical (up-and-down) movement of bouncing on a rebounder. The acceleration and the deceleration that come from bouncing create pressure changes within the body, and an increased amount of weight against the cell membranes, stimulating and strengthening them. All the movement provides a kind of cellular massage, which increases circulation, opens blood vessels and breaks up blockages, improves drainage of the lymph, and strengthens the cell membrane. Your whole body, not just your muscles, gets toned, cleansed, and strengthened—on a cellular level, from the inside out. That's why both Shelley and I do it every day.

Rebounding is the most convenient, metabolically effective, acid-removing form of exercise I know. It strengthens the entire body, increases circulation, improves digestion and elimination, protects the heart, supports the endocrine system and adrenal glands, improves thyroid function, eases menstrual problems, strengthens muscles, improves bone density, releases stress, pumps the lymphatic system, promotes cell growth and repair, improves the immune system, fights disease processes, and reverses the symptoms of aging. What more could you ask for in a form of exercise?

How about: Rebounding reduces body fat levels; firms legs, thighs, abdomens, arms, and hips; increases agility; improves balance; builds endurance; and increases energy levels. It also improves your performance in an array of other athletic endeavors. And all this it does without the stress of impact that attends so many other forms of exercise. Rebounding stimulates the metabolism, burns calories effectively, and more important removes acids through the skin and elimination organs. Rebounding fights obesity!

Rebounding is the best way I know to simultaneously reduce acidic body fat and firm body tissues with aerobic exercise.

Total Calories Spent Per Minute of Jogging on the Health Rebounder

Body Weight (pounds)	Calories spent (minutes)				
	1	5	10	15	20
90	2.9	14.5	29.0	43.5	58.0
100	3.4	17.0	34.0	51.0	68.0
110	3.9	19.5	39.0	58.5	78.0
120	4.4	22.0	44.0	66.0	88.0
130	4.9	24.5	49.0	73.5	98.0
140	5.4	27.0	54.0	81.0	108.0
150	6.0	30.0	60.0	90.0	120.0
160	6.5	32.5	65.0	97.5	130.0
170	7.0	35.0	70.0	105.0	140.0
180	7.5	37.5	75.0	112.5	150.0
190	8.0	40.0	80.0	120.0	160.0

On the rebounder, you bounce up and down against gravity. Because you're not landing on solid ground, there's no trauma to the joints. Working against the constant gravitational pressure, alternating weightlessness at the top of the bounce and double-gravity at the bottom, rebounding produces a pumping action that pulls acidic waste products out of the cells and forces oxygen and other nutrients from the bloodstream into them. This provides a number of benefits; I'll detail a few of the key ones here:

Rebounding is good for your heart. You can, of course, attain your target heart rate while rebounding. The aerobic effect of rebounding often surpasses that of running. (See chart on page 155.) Beyond that, rebounding strengthens your heart in two ways. It improves the tone and quality of the muscle itself, and it increases the coordination of the muscle fibers as they drain blood out of the heart during each beat. Rebounding can also lower cholesterol and triglyceride levels by removing excess acid, and lower blood pressure. And it allows the heart to beat less often when at rest, meaning your heart is running easily and efficiently. Regular rebounding, at least fifteen minutes five days a week, protects you against heart disease.

Rebounding is detoxifying. The movement of rebounding stimulates the lymphatic system, helping it drain away the body's metabolic wastes, ridding you of acidic toxins and other junk cast off by cells. The lymphatic system does not have its own pump, the way the circulation system has the heart. There are just three ways to move the fluid around through the lymph vessels: gravitational pressure, lymphatic massage—and the muscular contraction from exercise and movement. Rebounding effectively provides all three.

Rebounding stabilizes the nervous system. Exercise is a great way to relieve stress. Rebounding has the additional benefit of the repetitive bouncing motion, which can put you into an almost trance-like state of total relaxation. It can be meditative, or hypnotic. You get the benefits not only while you're bouncing, but also continuing into your whole lifestyle. You'll be more resistant to environmental, physical, emotional, and mental stress. My clients who rebound tell me they can think better, work longer, and learn more easily. They also say they relax more easily, sleep better, and feel less tense and nervous. They report that the exercise invigorates them and fills them with a sense of well-being.

Rebounding builds muscle. Rebounding allows the muscles to go through their full range of motion with equal force, the best way to produce true physical strength, according to James White, Ph.D., director of research in rehabilitation in the physical education department at the University of California at San Diego. Rebounding improves the coordination of nerve impulse transmission to muscle fibers, meaning the muscles can work more effectively and efficiently. And it increases muscle fiber tone, which creates muscular strength. As Dr. White points out, rebounding also helps you learn to shift your weight properly, be aware of the position of your body, and improve your balance, which is not only good for you all around but also lets you *use* the strength you have.

All these benefits are there for anyone who rebounds for at least fifteen minutes at least five times a week. Just about anyone can rebound. It's good for all ages—a form of exercise you can enjoy for a lifetime. Rebounding can be adjusted to meet your current fitness level, then move you up from there. You easily control the intensity of the workout, depending on how vigorously you bounce and how high you lift your feet off the mat. Rebounding is safe, convenient, and inexpensive. It provides the ideal aerobic effect, without exhausting you or depriving your cells of sufficient oxygen. Quite simply, it is one of the most effective forms of motion known. Plus, it is *fun* to bounce!

Rebounding vs. Other Exercise

Most other forms of exercise apply weight to specific muscles or groups of muscles, but rebounding targets every single cell in your body at once, applying pressure nearly one hundred times a minute. Other forms of exercise, including weight lifting and many calisthenics like push-ups, pull-ups, and sit-ups, use a repetitive up-and-down motion

the way rebounding does, but these conventional exercises still isolate specific muscles or muscle groups. That makes it very time con-
suming to work out the whole body, for one thing, as well as
stressing the body much more than rebounding requires in an attempt to reach the same goal. It also increases the opportunity for
injury. You could get many of the benefits of rebounding by jumping
rope, but you'd be courting joint and back pain from all that slam-
ming down on the ground with the full force of your body—aided by
gravity. Moreover, jumping rope won't pump the lymphatic system
the way rebounding does. In general, rebounding is more effective
for both fitness and weight loss than cycling, running, or jogging, according to Dr. White, with the added advantage of producing dramatically fewer injuries (over both the short and long term). NASA
research determined that rebounding is a 68 percent more effective
aerobic exercise than jogging.

Another thing that sets rebounding apart from the most common forms of exercise like jogging, walking, biking, and weight lifting is that it provides isotonic, isometric, calisthenic, and aerobic
exercise all in one go. It lets you tone specific muscles by moving
them with a constant load applied, as in weight lifting (isotonic exercise). You can isolate specific muscles or muscle groups to focus on
by creating muscular contractions without movement of the body
part involved (isometric exercise). And you can activate the body's
largest, most powerful muscles with small, gentle, precise motions
consistently applied to quickly tighten and tone those areas (calisthenic exercise).

And you do all this aerobically. As you'll see in the descriptions
and illustrations of different rebounding techniques that follow, you
can target every part of the body with rebounding, including the
thighs, knees, hips, buttocks, waist, stomach, and arms. Bouncing,
jumping, jogging, kicking, and twisting in place on the rebounder is
a full-body weight-bearing activity that strengthens muscles, con-
nective tissue, ligaments, and bones. Changing the angle of the body
changes the stress on the muscles—leaning back as you kick your
legs places more stress on the stomach muscles; leaning forward
as you lift your legs behind you puts more stress on your glutes—
making different cells work against gravity, which tightens, lifts, and

tones the muscles and even the organs and skin. Plus, fifteen minutes a day is enough to challenge every cell in your cardiovascular pulmonary system to be all that it can be.

Total Calories Burned: Rebounding vs. Jogging

Body Weight (pounds)	Calories Burned	
	Jogging 1 mile (12 minutes at 5 mph)	Rebounding (12 minutes)
100	47	58
105	49	60
110	52	63
115	54	65
120	56	67
125	59	70
130	61	72
135	64	75
140	66	77
145	68	79
150	71	82
155	73	84
160	75	86
165	78	89
170	80	91
175	82	93
180	85	96
185	87	98
190	89	100
195	92	103
200	94	105

This chart comes from the research performed by Victor L. Katch, Ph.D., Department of Physical Education, University of Michigan at Ann Arbor.

THE RIGHT REBOUNDER

A rebounder is just a small, low-slung trampoline with a strong woven mat attached by coiled steel springs to a steel frame with six legs 7 to 9 inches long. (Spring-loaded legs allow for easy folding and storage of the rebounder.) Most are round, though you can also find rectangular, square, or polygonal rebounders. The jumping surface is typically 28 inches in diameter. On most models you can add an optional stabilizing bar for anyone who needs or wants something to hold on to to steady themselves, for a greater sense of security as they bounce. These bars attach to two of the frame's legs and reach roughly waist high.

Rebounders are fairly cheap, but beware, as the lowest-cost models are often nothing more than toys. Bouncing on poorly constructed models, usually imported from Asia, can be harmful to one's muscles, nerves, joints, and tendons. There's no yield to them, and the abrupt jarring effect is not much different from landing on the floor. As with so many things in life, you get what you pay for. If you can possibly afford it, go for a more top-of-the-line model from a sporting goods store, department store, catalog, or health food store. Buying direct from the manufacturer if possible will probably get you the best price. (See Resources.) In any case, a good rebounder will still cost less than a year's membership at most gyms. And a rebounder should last for many years.

A key feature to look for is how the net/mat is constructed. The material shouldn't stretch at all during the downward landing—the springs should be doing all the work there—and provide a resilient rebound. Such a mat will be made from Permatron material, which has a smooth finish. Permatron is resistant to ultraviolet rays and doesn't absorb moisture, and so won't break down like other fabrics. The mat should be sewn together with 6,000 stitches of high-grade nylon thread, with two layers of strong polypropylene webbing stitched around the edge.

The frame should be heavy-grade steel attached to the mat by thirty-six 4-inch-long springs made of quality wire to deliver a soft bounce. The springs should be shielded by a protective cover. Individual spring mounting pens prevent frame wear. Tapered coils generally last longer; tube coils that aren't tapered in low-quality springs require frequent replacement. That's another point to consider: Replacement springs should be available directly from the manufacturer; retail distributors rarely stock them. The legs of the rebounder should fold easily so you can store it under a bed or behind a door. You can buy a travel rebounder; its frame should fold in half and come with a carrying bag.

No one manufacturer has cornered the market on quality rebounders. One device that exhibits all the features of excellence I've been describing here are the Needak Health Rebounders, available in the original vigorous rebounding class unit, the soft bounce rebounder, and the travel model, all of which come with an optional, easily attached stabilizing bar.

How Much Is Enough?

One great thing about the pH Miracle Living view of exercise is that you must also ask: How much is too much? One reason this program works for everyone is that anyone can do it. That includes the exercise component. Any person at any skill level can start this program and benefit immediately. And because it takes just fifteen minutes a day, any schedule can accommodate it. Even yours! And you don't want to over-exercise, at the risk of acidifying rather than alkalinizing your body.

This program gives you 15 minutes a day, 5 days a week, on your rebounder, a full program for complete fitness. You could do this up to 7 days a week, 2 to 3 times a day if you so desire, though beyond that you'd be over-exercising. If you don't exercise every day, acids will build up in your tissues—and you will gain weight! To get an equivalent workout without rebounding, I suggest a 30- to 45-minute walk or jog over hilly terrain. Whatever exercise you do, make sure it is helpfully and healthfully aerobic. You must get to the point where you break a sweat within 10 to 15 minutes. With rebounding, you should be sweating by midway through the aerobic section of the workout, around the 5- to 10-minute mark. You've got to sweat to receive the maximum benefits of exercising.

All these time frames rely on you taking in an appropriate amount of food (calories/electrons) each day. If you're eating more than you should, you'll need to exercise longer to discourage the excess from collecting in your body's fat stores. That's why you'll find so much conflicting advice out there about just how much exercise you need. Experts can't seem to agree on whether or not they should account for Americans' well-established habit of eating too much when they make declarations about how much exercise is ideal. If you're following the pH Miracle Living eating plan, however, I know your body is getting the fuel it needs—no more, no less—and so you can streamline your workout accordingly.

Building Muscle

Rebounding will strengthen you, as noted earlier. I do recommend an additional set of exercises to target specific muscles. I'll tell you how to do the actual exercises a little later in this chapter, but for now I just want to explain the general technique and the theory behind it. I'm going to do *that* because unless you really understand the process, you won't believe that it will work.

Here's what you do for a full body workout: Do 8 exercises. For each of 8 exercises, do one (1) repetition. At the point where your muscle is fully flexed, hold for at least 15 (and no more than 30) seconds. Return to the starting position—and go on to the next exercise. Do this 3 times each week, and that's it. Eight exercises, 1 time, for a total of roughly 2 minutes, and you're done. Actually, make that 4 minutes, since you should bounce on the rebounder for 15 seconds after you finish each move.

Here's why this radical approach not only works, but works better than any other technique. The whole idea is to stimulate contractions of and blood flow to the specific muscles you wish to increase

Jeffrey

I'm thirty-five and have been doing this program for about a year. I took off over 50 pounds in the first twelve weeks! I've gone from about 320 pounds to under 215; from a 48-inch waist to 36; from an XXXL T-shirt to a plain old L. I wake up full of en-

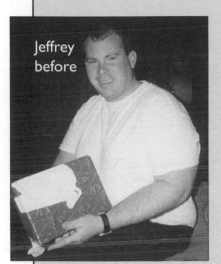

Jeffrey
before

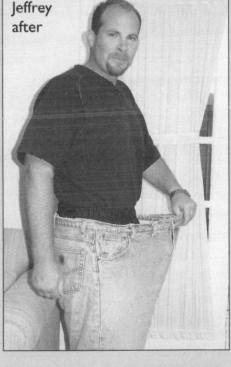

Jeffrey
after

ergy and no longer have a "down" time in the early afternoon. I'm exercising and totally enjoying it. And, both my children are eating extremely well.

When I first really learned about this program, I was completely blown away. I immediately began to make small, comfortable changes, then started using the green drink with pH drops. Before that, my diet consisted of pizza, pasta, beer, caffeinated soda, huge burgers, and fried foods of all kinds. I considered "vegetable" a four-letter word. Of course, I knew that continuing to eat in such a fashion would eventually end my life, but I also thought of "diet" as a four-letter word. Putting any kind of effort toward losing weight was just not in my game plan.

All that changed when I found something that made sense to me. I'm working now to change my health on a cellular level. When I put food in my mouth, I sometimes find myself thinking, "Will this help me or hurt me?" or "Will this food energize me or slow me down?" These are very different questions from last year, when my thoughts were more like "Pepperoni or sausage?" or "Fries with that?"!

in size and strength. Flexing the muscle creates a positively charged site, and this attracts blood, which is negatively charged. These opposite charges create circulation directly to the muscle being exercised. The creation of this electromagnetic attraction of blood to muscle begins the strengthening and increasing size of the muscle, as the red blood cells are biologically transformed into muscle cells. When weight or stress is applied to a muscle, it applies weight or pressure against the cell membranes, causing increased blood flow. When the blood arrives in the muscle, it not only supplies electron-rich oxygen, but also begins to change back into an embryonic cell and then gradually into a muscle cell, according to the principles of New Biology (explained in more detail in *The pH Miracle*).

What makes this technique so effective is the fact that the blood pools in the muscle for a longer period rather than moving quickly in and out the way it does in the more familiar "3 sets of 15 reps" workout format. So the muscle is built not only better but also more quickly. It is important, however, to "bounce out" on the rebounder any residual acid created in this process, as you'll see in the following directions.

THE REBOUND WORKOUT

In this section, I'm going to outline basic exercises you can do on your rebounder. At the end of the chapter, I'll tell you how to put them all together and combine with the weight lifting described earlier to create The pH Miracle Living exercise plan. The exercises appear here in roughly the order you should use them: first the warm-up and stretches, next the aerobic components, and finally the exercises targeting specific muscles or muscle groups.

Soft bounce. This is the way you should warm up and the motion you should use as you transition between other exercises described here. Stand in the center of the rebounder with your feet hip-width apart. Keeping your back straight, your knees just slightly bent, and your arms down by your side or on your hips, bounce up and down gently, without your feet leaving the mat. Your toes and calf muscles power the motion.

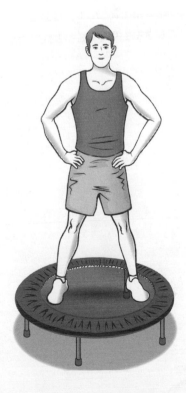

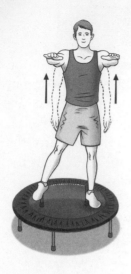

Tap out. From a soft bounce with your feet near the outside edges of the mat, shift your weight onto one leg and tap the other foot to the outer edge of the mat. At the same time, raise your arms straight in front of you until they are parallel with the ground. Lower your arms, then raise them again as you shift to the other side.

Jumping jack. This is a high-bounce exercise, meaning your feet come up off the mat as you bounce. This, too, should be a familiar motion. Start in the center of the rebounder with your feet together and your hands at your sides. Jump up and land with your feet on opposite edges of the rebounder mat while swinging your arms out to the side and up overhead. Jump again and return to the start position. This is great for your calves, quadriceps, hamstrings, buttocks, abdominals, arms, and shoulders.

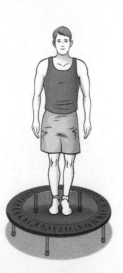
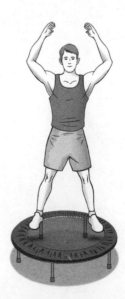

Hamstring and buttocks curl. From a soft bounce, shift your weight to one leg and lift the other behind you, bent at the knee, with your foot aiming toward your buttocks. At the same time, extend both arms behind you, palms facing into your body (a reverse triceps curl). Lower your arms and leg, then repeat on the other side. Lean slightly forward as you lift your legs behind you. Make sure you feel your buttocks and triceps tightening.

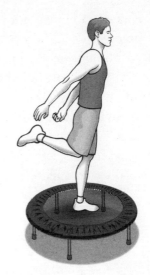

Walking/jogging. This aerobic exercise increases cardiovascular and lymphatic circulation. It should be fairly self-explanatory. Starting in the center of the rebounder, perform a walking, jogging, or sprinting motion, lifting your knees high in front of you. Proceed at your own speed; don't wait for the rebounder to bounce your leg up.

Begin by doing 50 bounces this way, building up to 100, 150, and finally 200. You should keep it up about 3 to 5 minutes.

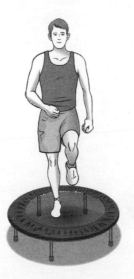
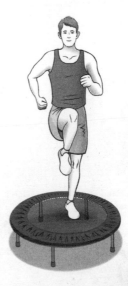

Variation: For an additional benefit, sprint as fast as you can for 25 bounces or 15 seconds, whichever comes first. Follow that with 10 soft bounces. Build up gradually to 100 "sprinting" bounces, pausing for 10 soft bounces after each set of 25. This provides an optimum workout for the cardiovascular system. In addition, it will give your buttocks, hamstrings, quadriceps, arms, and abdominals an extreme workout. Make sure you return to the soft bounce for at least 15 seconds after this or any isometric or isotonic exercise to remove any lactic acid buildup.

Hand to knee. Jog easily, alternating tapping the right knee with the left hand and the left knee with the right hand. This exercise helps coordination and balance while working the entire body.

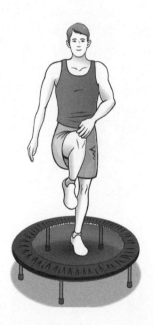

Elbow to knee. Bounce and bring the right knee up to meet the left elbow. Then bounce once on both feet before raising the left knee to touch the right elbow. Continue alternating sides with a two-footed bounce in between each side. This is another excellent exercise for balance and coordination.

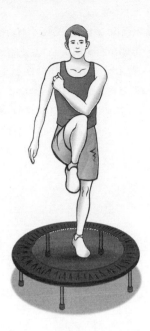

Hand to heel. Bounce and bring your right leg behind you and tap your heel with your left hand. Bounce on both feet, then do the opposite side. Continue alternating. This is one more excellent exercise for balance and coordination.

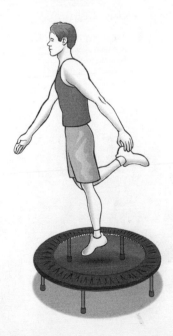

High bounce. An all-body exercise. Start standing naturally in the center of the rebounder. Bend your knees and use your calves and toes to bounce up off the mat (clearing 4 to 10 inches), and land again in the same spot. You can do this exercise with your arms down by your sides or extended over your head.

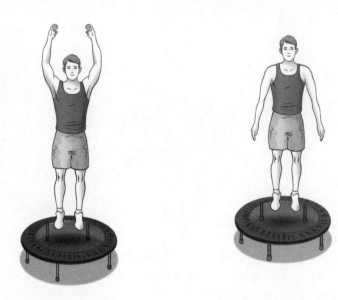

Knee-high sprints. Jog briskly, lifting your knees as high as possible. This excellent aerobic exercise works the entire body.

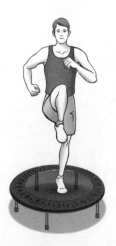

Triceps curl. With the feet together, and the knees slightly bent, bounce gently on the balls of your feet, leaning forward about 10 degrees, and do a reverse triceps curl by extending both arms behind you, palms facing into your body. Your feet should come off the mat as you bounce. This simple motion works the calves, quadriceps, hamstrings, buttocks, triceps, and abdominals.

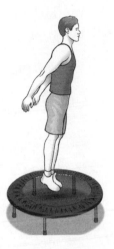

Upright row. This exercise works your chest, abdominals, upper arms, shoulders, calves, quadriceps, hamstrings, and buttocks. From a soft bounce, shift your weight to one side and lift the other knee

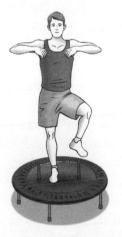
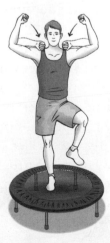

until your thigh is almost parallel to the floor, then switch legs: it's basically a marching motion. Your arms start at your sides, then pull up, with your elbows out to the side, until your hands are in front of your chest, in a rowing gesture. Return your arms to your sides.

If you wish, use this exercise as part of your stretching bounce before the aerobic/cardio portion of your workout.

Variation: Using the same leg motions, raise your arms over your head, then lower your fists, thumbs down, to your shoulders, with your elbows out to the side; raise to start.

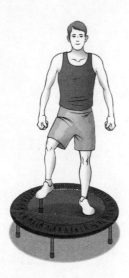

The side to side. This is a great exercise for the thighs, hips, and stomach. Stand with your feet slightly wider than hip-width apart and your arms in front of you, not quite completely extended, with your hands about hip-high. Move from side to side in a soft bounce, shifting your weight from foot to foot in a fluid, rhythmic motion. Beginners should keep their feet on the mat; in more advanced versions the feet can leave the mat in turn.

This is a great transition exercise out of your soft bounce warm-up.

The slalom. Start to the right of center of the mat, with your legs together and your feet parallel, toes pointing ahead and to the left. Bounce, with your feet coming up off the mat, and shift position so that you land to the left of center, with your toes pointing ahead and to the right. Repeat, alternating sides. Your knees and hips should be bent slightly, like a skier. All the action is below the hips, while the upper body remains virtually motionless, facing straight ahead. Keep your back straight and stay on the balls of your feet. This exercise is great for coordination and strengthening of the calves and quads and the muscles in the torso, particularly the hips. It also isolates the hamstrings, buttocks, and abdominals. It's an excellent way to improve your balance. If you choose to use hand weights during this exercise, hold them as you would ski poles!

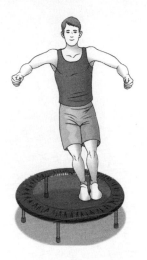

The washing machine. Starting in the middle of the rebounder, bounce and turn your hips and legs to the left and your chest and shoulders to the right. Your right arm extends out to your side at shoulder level, while the left, at the same level, bends in so your fist is in front of your chest and your elbow points out to the side. On the next bounce, shift position so your hips and legs go right and your chest, shoulders, and arms go left. Continue alternating sides. Keep your back straight and your knees slightly bent. (To decrease intensity, don't raise your arms as high.) This works the calves, quads, hamstrings, buttocks, abdominals, shoulders, and biceps. This move is great for the waistline and digestion.

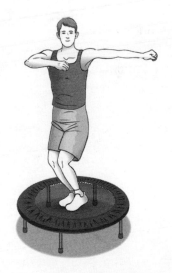

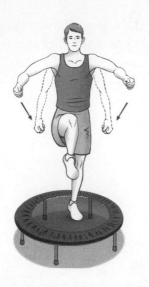

Forward knee lift. Bouncing in the center of the rebounder, raise one knee to waist height so your thigh is parallel to the floor, while your arms move as if you are holding a tray you're going to break across the raised knee. Beginners should keep the other foot on the mat; more advanced rebounders should let the "standing" foot leave the mat as they bounce. This exercise focuses on the calves, quadriceps, buttocks, hamstrings, abdominals, chest, arms, and shoulders.

Abdominal bounce. This exercise focuses on the glutes and abs. In each of the several variations targeting your abdominal muscles, you actually bounce on your buttocks, with your legs either on the ground or in the air.

Variation 1: For beginners. Bounce with your back straight up (perpendicular to the floor), your legs bent so your feet are flat on the floor, and your hands resting on the rim of the rebounder. Once you've mastered that, lean back to 45 degrees, but leave your feet on the floor. Increase the difficulty by lifting one leg and then the other while you bounce, and/or by placing your hands behind your head.

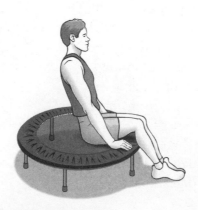

Variation 2: Advanced. Sit in the middle of the rebounder, lean back to a 45-degree angle, and lift your legs to a 45-degree angle, so your body makes a "V" shape. Bounce on your butt without touching the rebounder with your hands, with your arms out in front of you as if you were holding the reins to a horse. Keep your eyes looking straight ahead, for balance, and squeeze the upper and lower abdominal muscles together as you bounce. This is a difficult, but most effective, way to do this exercise. Increase the challenge by pumping your arms up and down (while still "holding the reins").

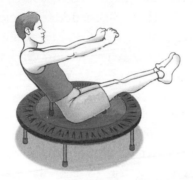

Variation 3: While in a modified "V" position, alternate your legs, while bouncing side to side, landing alternately on your left and right buttocks. Bounce first with one leg straight and extended out, parallel to the floor or slightly elevated, and the other bent and pulled in toward your chest. Then, as you extend the bent leg, pull in the extended leg; keep alternating. Increase the difficulty by doing a full abdominal crunch, bringing both legs in to your chest, knees first, then extending them out fully again, returning to the "V" position.

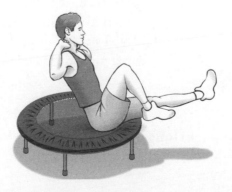

WEIGHTS WORKOUT

If you've ever done any weight lifting, these movements (if not the technique) will no doubt already be familiar to you. You need to do only 1 rep of each exercise. That's right: one set of one rep! This is the most efficient and effective muscle-building technique available. And it is very simple—even someone who has never picked up a weight before can do it. But trust me when I tell you, it isn't as easy to do as it sounds!

Use the maximum amount of weight you can hold at the point of greatest resistance for 15 to 30 seconds. If you can't hold it for 15 seconds, then decrease the weight. When you can hold it for longer than 30 seconds, then increase the weight. You don't need very heavy weights. I start with 20 pounds in each hand when I'm working my arms, for example. You may find that you need different amounts of weight for different exercises.

After completing each exercise, take a deep breath in through your nose and breathe it out through your mouth. Then do the soft bounce on the rebounder for 15 seconds to get rid of any acid buildup in the muscle being stressed.

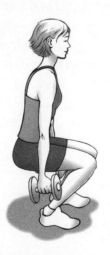

Dumbbell squats. This exercise works your thighs. Stand with your feet slightly wider than your shoulders and angled outward. Holding a dumbbell in each hand, with your arms down along your sides and your palms facing your thighs, bend your knees until your thighs are parallel to the ground. Keep your back flat and your head up. Hold, then return, slowly and with good control, to start position.

Reverse (step-back) lunge. This exercise works the back of your thighs. Stand with your feet hip-width apart with your arms along your sides with a weight in each hand. Step one foot behind you and bend both knees, lowering your torso (keeping it straight!) toward the ground until your front thigh is parallel to the ground and your back thigh is perpendicular to it. Hold, then slowly rise and step your feet back together.

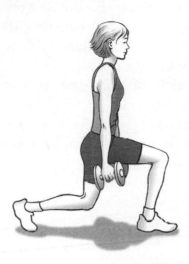

Dumbbell bench press. This exercise works your back. Lie on your back on the floor, or, better still, on a bench press bench. With a weight in each hand (or, using a barbell if you have one), begin with your arms raised straight up toward the ceiling from your shoulders, with your hands slightly closer together than your shoulders. Under very strict control, lower the weights toward the upper part of your chest, bending your elbows out to the sides. Pause briefly, then begin

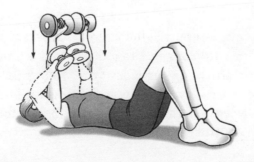

to raise up again until you find the point of most resistance, about halfway up, with your elbows still bent. Hold there. Then slowly return to the starting position, with your arms straight.

Two-arm dumbbell rows. This exercise works your back. Sit on the floor, leaning back at a 45-degree angle, with your legs straight out in front of you, or bent at the knee with your feet flat on the floor. Extend your arms in front of you, parallel to the floor at shoulder height, with a weight in each hand. Your palms can face each other, or face down to the floor.

Row the dumbbell toward your chest—it should break the plain of the torso slightly—and hold. Return to start position with good control.

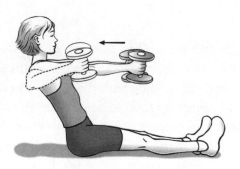

Dumbbell side laterals. This exercise works your shoulders. Stand up straight with your feet together. Hold a dumbbell in each hand, with your arms at your sides with your palms facing your thighs. Raise your arms straight out to the side until they are parallel to the ground. Keep a slight bend in your elbow. Hold, then lower slowly and with control to the start position.

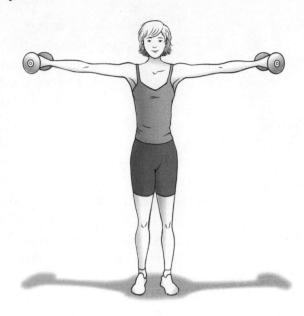

Dumbbell curls. This exercise works the biceps in your arms. Stand with your feet hip-width apart with a dumbbell in each hand and your arms down in front of your body with your palms facing forward, away from your body. Keeping your elbows tucked in at your waist, curl the weights forward and up toward your chest. Do not use any sudden jerking, yanking, or thrusting to get the motion started; it should be a smooth continuous motion. Pause briefly at the top and lower with good control until you reach the point of greatest resistance and hold. Your arm and chest muscles should be fully flexed. Then return slowly to the start position.

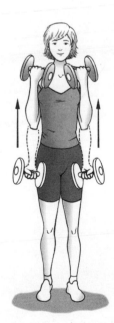

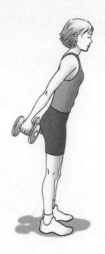

Dumbbell triceps extension. This exercise works the triceps in your arms. Stand with your feet apart and lean slightly forward, keeping your back straight and your arms along your sides with a weight in each hand. Your palms should face behind you or, for a slightly different feeling, toward your thighs. Raise your straight arms directly behind you, away from your body, as high as you can. Hold at the top of the arc, then return slowly to the start position.

Standing calf raise. This exercise works your calves. Stand with your feet hip-width apart with a weight in each hand and your arms straight alongside you. Lift up off your heels onto the balls of your feet as high as you can. Hold, then lower slowly back to the ground.

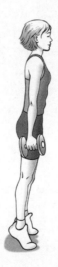

THE PH MIRACLE LIVING WORKOUT

The pH Miracle Living workout has two somewhat different phases you do on alternating days.

1. You're going to do 15 minutes on the rebounder every day, or at least 5 times a week.
2. Three days a week (not consecutive days), you're going to add in the 8 weight-lifting exercises.

And on Sunday, you rest. Your body needs that too!

Warm-up. Begin each workout with a warm-up.

- Do the **soft bounce** for 2 minutes to increase blood flow and get everything moving, preparing your body for the work ahead.
- The **tap out** and the **side to side** are also good for warming up.

BREATHE

If you like you can add this deep-breathing exercise to your warm-up to increase the alkalizing of your body: Start standing with your arms at your sides. Lift your arms out to the sides and up over your head, keeping your palms facing up so they eventually touch over your head. Take a deep breath through your nose as you raise your arms up and out to the side. As they reach shoulder high, continue breathing in, but now through your mouth and continue raising your arms until your palms touch up over your head. As you do this you should feel oxygen going deep into your lungs. Let your breath out through your mouth, slowly, as you return your arms to your sides. You may want to hold your breath for a count of 4 while your arms are overhead and your lungs are full of oxygen before releasing your breath and your arms. Breathing out through the mouth prolongs the exhalation, helping to release the air that is generally left in the lungs when you are breathing shallowly—air that contains more acidic carbon dioxide—and replacing it with fresh alkalizing air containing more oxygen.

You can do this breathing exercise on or off the rebounder (though it only counts as warm-up if you bounce while doing it!). I recommend doing this every day, 10 to 15 times. It will begin the process of feeding oxygen to the whole body, and especially the brain, increasing circulation and improving cognitive function—and keeping you alkaline and slim!

Stretch. The next phase is a 2-minute stretch, while doing a soft bounce with your feet shoulder-width apart.

- For the first stretch, reach both arms overhead and stretch as high as you can. Lean left and then right for 25 bounces.

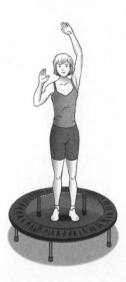

- Second, reach your right arm up toward the sky alongside your head, then bend it at the elbow and send your hand down behind your head and neck. Use your right hand to gently stretch your left arm behind your head, holding for 5 seconds, or about 3 bounces. Then switch arms.

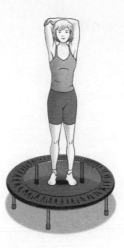

- For the third stretch, extend your right arm across your chest, gently pulling your upper arm in toward you with the left hand. Hold for about 5 seconds, or about 3 bounces. Do the other arm in the same way. For a more advanced stretch, alternate kicking your legs out, in front and/or behind you.

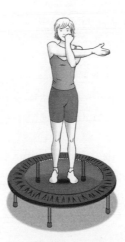

- You can also use the **upright row**, the **jumping jack**, the **tap out**, the **side to side**, and the **hamstring and buttocks curl** as part of your 2 minutes of stretching.

Weights. On the days you are doing the weight-lifting exercises described above, they should come next. You can do them on or off the rebounder, but be sure to bounce for 15 seconds between each exercise either way.

Rebounder. Every day (or at least 5 times a week) you need to run through the rebounder exercises described in this chapter. This too is divided into two parts. First the cardio conditioning portion, followed by the isometric portion targeting specific muscles (other than the heart!).

1. You should spend 5 minutes concentrating on aerobics, running, jogging or walking in place, and/or doing the **high bounce, knee-high sprints**, or **jumping jacks**.

Jog or run in place for at least 200 bounces. For whatever time remains, mix in other exercises if you wish, building up from 25 bounces of any given one to up to 100. For each isometric rebounding exercise, begin by doing one set of 25 bounces of each before moving on to the next exercise. Once you've mastered that, work up to 50 bounces, then eventually 75, and finally 100. Try to increase each week, so that after 4 weeks you are up to the total of 100, though you can set a different pace for yourself if you want or need to. Also, you might be ready for more repetitions of some moves sooner than others, and that's okay. As long as you are rebounding for your 15 minutes a day, you're benefiting.

2. Spend another 5 minutes working different specific parts of the body with a series including some or all of the following:

- Forward knee lift
- Hand to knee
- Elbow to knee
- Hand to heel
- Knee-high sprints
- Hamstring and buttocks curl
- Triceps curl

- Upright row
- Washing machine
- Slalom
- Abdominal exercises (but save them for last)

If you can't fit all the exercises into the time allotted, and you don't want to run over, do the ones that zero in on the areas of your body that need the most work. Or do the ones you think are the most fun! Do be sure to get in the abdominals every time, though, at least 25 bounces of each variation you do.

Cool down. The final phase of each workout is to cool down by doing the soft bounce for 1 minute. This is another good time to do the deep-breathing exercise, if you so choose.

THE pH MIRACLE LIVING WORKOUT AT A GLANCE

- Warm-up: 2 minutes
- Stretch: 2 minutes
- Weight lifting: 4 minutes (3x/week)
- Aerobic/cardio rebounding: 5 minutes
- Isometric rebounding: 5 minutes, including, lastly, an abdominal bounce for at least 25 bounces
- Cool down: 1 minute

PUMP UP THE PROGRAM

Once you've mastered the basic pH Miracle Living workout, there are a couple of ways you can increase the intensity of the workout. These are always optional; the basic program is enough to keep anyone at a healthy weight. But for those who want to develop their muscles more precisely, or amp up the workout, or just have a change of pace, here are some options:

Using weights on the rebounder. You can increase resistance by using hand or ankle weights for any or all parts of your rebounding workout. The force of gravity increases the weight one and a half times as you contact the mat, so this is a very powerful way to increase size and strength of muscles quickly. But you'll need to use very light weights. Start with 1-pound weights, working up (if you can or want to) to 2 or maybe 2½ pounds. Even if you move up on some exercises, lower weights might still be best for others. I generally use 2½ pounds, for example, but just 1 pound when I'm doing jumping jacks. If you do use weights on the rebounder, I suggest starting out with weights for 25 bounces at first, working up by sets of 25 until you can do all 100 bounces with the weights. If you want to increase the weight, do so gradually, and only after you've mastered doing all 100 bounces with the original weight.

You can also do your eight weight-lifting exercises on the rebounder if you so desire, while doing a soft bounce. Use your regular weight dumbbells for this purpose. Alternately, if you use light dumbbells for most or all of your regular rebound workout, you can skip the extra weight lifting altogether and complete your entire workout every day in just 15 minutes.

Plyometric jumping. This means increasing intensity by increasing speed. That is, do whatever you were already doing—but faster! This allows you to improve your coordination and agility, which decreases your risk of injury, as well as intensify your aerobic workout. Start by doing one or two movements in your regular routine rapidly, and master them before adding more, one by one. You can start by doing just a portion of the bounces of each exercise rapidly, and work up to doing the whole set that way.

Ryan

I was very unhappy with the way my body was looking, so I entered a fitness and weight-loss contest connected to a best-selling book. I was very dedicated, but I just wasn't having any success. Then I switched to the pH Miracle program and lost 31 pounds of fat while gaining 11 pounds of muscle—in just twelve weeks! I went on to be one of the top winners in that original contest, even beating the last year's grand champion. All without meat, chicken, or protein drinks, building muscle with blood and building blood with green foods and green drinks.

EXERCISING SAFELY

You've already learned the most important safety tip when it comes to exercising safely, efficiently, and effectively: Do it in a way that will alkalize, rather than acidify, your body. Besides that, here are a few basic tips on integrating exercise into your life in a wholly beneficial way.

- Keep hydrating. You need even more water (or green drink) while you exercise.
- Start slow and work up gradually to the full program. This is especially important if you haven't been active, but it also applies when you are already active but beginning a new form of exercise. Begin with lower weights and work up from there. Start with fewer reps and build up. Begin by just doing the soft bounce and work up to more complicated jumps. Or rebound for shorter periods until you are ready for the full 15 minutes.
- Use the support bar anytime you are doing a new or complicated bounce, especially anything that involves moving your legs out away from your body. As your strength and balance improve you may find you don't need the bar.
- Avoid overly rigorous workouts. More is not always better!
- Don't exercise when you are very ill. Sometimes, your body needs rest more than it needs exercise. When you start to

feel your energy coming back, by all means continue with your regular program, even if you need to modify it temporarily.
- Consult with your health care provider before beginning this or any exercise program.

SWEAT MORE, WEIGH LESS

If you are exercising moderately but not sweating, or not sweating much, try the following strategies to get the acids flowing from your body:

- Make sure you are drinking the amount of water recommended in chapter 5. Build up to it gradually if necessary.
- Drink at least 1 liter of green drink at least 30 minutes before exercising.
- Exercise more often or for longer periods of time. Do 30 minutes instead of 15, or do your 15-minute routine twice a day. In general, more often is better than longer.
- If you can't exercise, you can still sweat: Take a 30-minute infrared dry heat sauna at 140 degrees Fahrenheit. Be sure to hydrate yourself with green drink. This kind of sauna is the best passive exercise you can get. It will increase blood circulation, begin the movement of lymphatic fluids, and increase your heart rate as if you were moving. And you will sweat!
- Dry-brush your skin daily to open pores. You can do this in the shower after a workout.
- Take an Epsom salts bath to open the pores and draw out acidic toxins.
- Have a lymphatic massage twice a week to move acids from the tissues through the lymphatic system.

My goal is to make this program as fun as it is effective, and I hope you'll enjoy rebounding as much as I do. If not, choose something else that interests you; exercise only works if you actually do it! One great thing about this program is that you'll get positive reinforcement right away as you watch your body start to tone and firm up, and the pounds come off as you lose excess acid through eating and exercising *right*—in just fifteen minutes a day!

Chapter 11

Take Seven: Steps to Your Ideal Weight

The first step to knowledge is to know that we are ignorant.
—LORD DAVID CECIL

It takes three to four months for the body to recycle all its blood cells. That is, every three or four months, you have an entirely new supply of blood cells. Consequently, twelve weeks on this program is enough to replace all or most of the blood you have now with blood cells at the peak of health. With healthy blood comes a healthy body—and a healthy body has no use for excess pounds. Live the pH Miracle for healthy weight loss and it will change not only your weight but also your life. Forever. You'll be, literally and figuratively, a different person three months from now.

Tens of thousands of men, women, and children have used the alkaline lifestyle to lose weight and keep it off—and be healthy and strong. You have to experience for yourself the difference in how you feel, think, and act to understand the depth of change it brings about in you.

Some of you will plunge right in, do this all out, and see amazing immediate results. If that's an approach you are truly comfortable with—it's a personality thing—then I say, go for it. Most people, however, benefit from a slower shift. If you are in the second category, then I recommend working through the first six steps laid out in this chapter gradually so that when you reach the seventh step—which is, as I explain later, really the beginning of your twelve weeks—you are 100 percent ready to do the program 100 percent. That's the best formula I know for 100 percent results that are 100 percent permanent. Your life will change just as surely one small step at a time as it does for those who leap first and ask questions later. And it's more likely to be a change that feels natural—a change you'll stick with. A change for life.

So this chapter walks you through putting together all the pieces laid out in this book: hydrating your body, eating right, exercising properly, taking your supplements, and cleaning up your emotional, psychological (goals), and spiritual (cleansing inside and out) self. Then, finally, you're truly ready to start. With Step 7 you'll begin with a Liquid Cleanse, transition into the full pH Miracle Living program, and journey to the new, lean, healthy, energetic you.

STEP 1. HYDRATE

Your first step toward your ideal weight must be, for all the reasons given in chapter 5, to fully hydrate your body. That's a simple enough place to start: Drink water! Good water, of course. Alkaline water (pH 9.5 or above). If you don't have a water machine that will do the job, buy distilled water and add to it sodium bicarbonate, sodium chlorite, or sodium silicate, as described in chapter 5.

You must commit to getting all the water your body needs to be healthy, and at a healthy weight. To that end, take a minute right now to figure out how much water you need, and plan how you're going to get it. Recording it all in the space at the end of this section will help you set, and stay on, your course.

Every day you need 1 liter of alkaline water for every 30 pounds you weigh. Thus a 210-pound person needs 7 liters a day, a 150-pound person needs 5, and so on. Write down *your* target daily alkaline water intake in the space at the end of this section.

Estimate how much water you actually drink each day right now. Count only alkaline water, not soda, fruit juice, coffee, or other sweetened, caffeinated, or carbonated liquids. Translate how much you drink into liters; 1 liter is roughly 34 ounces, 1 cup is 8 ounces. Write this down in the space provided in the chart on page 193. Now calculate how much *more* you need to drink each day to reach your target, and note that down too.

Work up to your target gradually. I suggest increasing the amount of alkaline water you drink a little bit each day over the course of a week: Divide the amount of water you're adding in by 7—the amount you'll increase each day for a week until you're on target—and create a schedule for yourself. Make it real: Write it down in the chart. Keep it with you, or post it where you'll see it often. Then *do it*.

For example, if you weigh 180 pounds, you need to get 6 liters of electron-rich alkaline water every day. If you already average 2½ liters a day (which would be pretty good by typical American standards!), you need to add in 3½ more. Divided by 7, that means half a liter a day over the next week. Tomorrow, drink 3 liters, the day after 3½, the next day 4, and so on. Your chart would look like this:

	Amount of Water to Add (liters)	Daily Target (liters)
Day 1	½	3
Day 2	½	3½
Day 3	½	4
Day 4	½	4½
Day 5	½	5
Day 6	½	5½
Day 7	½	6

If the amount you calculated seems like too much to add each day, you can stretch out the time it takes to reach your target, over ten days or two weeks or whatever you think you need. If you do that, your progress may not be as rapid. But this is a lifetime plan, and taking the time to do it right in a way that is comfortable for you makes it more likely you'll stick with it and succeed over the long term. Of course, "gradual" isn't for everyone either; if you are one of these, go ahead and drink your target amount today! If your body reacts too strongly, you can always cut back and build up again slowly.

I realize this will seem like a lot to drink at first. And it will be a big change for most people. It might be helpful to schedule your intake, at least at first: 1 liter first thing in the morning, another at 10 A.M., another with lunch, and so on, throughout the day, with a final liter before bed. (Once again: Commit to it by writing it down!) You should have alkaline water on hand at all times. Once you begin, you'll find that the more water you provide your body, the more water it needs—and the more water you'll want. You'll develop the habit, and you won't have to think much about it anymore. You'll crave water.

If you come to a place where this plan stops working for you, where you've stopped losing weight but are not yet at your ideal healthy weight, then the first thing you should do is check your hydration level. When clients stop getting the results they want, or hit a plateau, it is almost always because they stopped doing the things that got them the results in the first place. Most often, they've stopped hydrating fully. When they go back to getting all the electron-rich alkaline water their bodies need, the pounds come off again. Subsequently, this first step on your path is also the first place to come back to should you ever lose your way.

The amount of water I need to drink each day (target):   _____ liters.

The amount of water I currently drink each day: _____ liters.

The amount of water I need to add to my day
(subtract the number on the second line from the number
on the first line):   _____ liters.

The amount of water I need to add each day over the
next week (divide the number above by 7):   _____ liters.

	Amount of Water to Add (liters)	Daily Target (liters)
Day 1		
Day 2		
Day 3		
Day 4		
Day 5		
Day 6		
Day 7		

STEP 2. EAT RIGHT FOR YOUR LIFE

Step 2 is eating whole, natural, unprocessed organic foods, building your diet around green vegetables and healthy fats, as described in chapters 8 and 6, respectively. This, too, you may want to do gradually, letting your body get accustomed to the new energy you will be providing, and getting rid of acids more slowly, with less chance of the unpleasant symptoms that can result from releasing toxins. Or go all out right away, if that's your style; the advice about building up to full hydration applies here as well.

For those who prefer the gradual approach, I call this period "transition." The transitioning process is covered in more detail in *The pH Miracle*. The "Transitioning" chapter in that book suggests twelve steps to eliminating acidic foods from your diet. Briefly, they are:

1. Rethink breakfast, ditching acidic cereals, eggs, baked goods, dairy products, fruit juice, and coffee in favor of the same alkaline foods you'd choose at other times of the day on this plan, especially green veggies.
2. Cover three-quarters of your plate at every meal with vegetables.
3. Increase the amount of your food you eat raw.
4. Phase out sugary desserts.
5. Eliminate meat.
6. Get off dairy products.
7. Cut out yeast.
8. Get rid of white flour.
9. Switch from white to brown rice.
10. Avoid added sugar.
11. Eat only low-sugar fruits.
12. Check your condiments.

Getting specific makes it sound like all you're doing is eliminating things you can eat, but by using the information about alkaline food in chapter 8, and the menus and recipes in chapter 12, you'll find healthy, alkaline alternatives at each turn. Some foods, like tofu or grains or pre-made veggie burgers or cooked foods, you might use more of during transition, but eventually cut down on or eliminate as your body becomes entirely alkaline.

Pam

When I first heard about the pH Miracle program from a trusted friend, a lot of it made sense to me. But I was sure I could never give up coffee, red meat, and beer. But I was in for quite a surprise!

It wasn't until some months later when I really decided to take control of my health. I had a lot of relatively little things that all together were seriously dragging me down, mainly poor sleep; circles and bags under my eyes; joint pain in my thumbs, left foot, and right knee; canker sores; menstrual cramps; and ADD [attention deficit disorder] (for which I was taking Ritalin). I had enough, so I thought I'd give the pH Miracle a try. Gradually, I began to make small changes to my diet. I believe that small changes are less traumatic and therefore, more long lasting. I substituted tortillas for bread, almond butter for peanut butter, and raw almonds for snack foods. I completely eliminated dairy. Avocados, which I love, became a staple of my diet.

As I made these small changes, I noticed small improvements in the way I felt. As I began to feel better, it got easier to make the next change. I switched from red meat to white meat. I began drinking 3 liters of green drink a day. After just 2 liters (on the first day), my body began to crave the greens! My body knew what was good for it. To my amazement, within three days, coffee began to taste too bitter to me. I went from a full pot of full-strength coffee each day to half a cup, and within a few weeks it was gone from my life altogether.

I have been drinking the greens for almost a year now, and I feel great. All my health challenges have vanished, or at least tremendously improved. I'm even sleeping through the night, every night, and not missing the Ritalin I no longer take. The absence of canker sores alone makes the entire journey worth it! Having witnessed the amazing changes in my body, even my husband and sons (six and eight) are now drinking the greens and slowly changing their diets as well. It's all enough to almost make me forget: I've lost 25 pounds!

STEP 3. EXERCISE

Step 3 involves getting the right kind of exercise, in the right amounts. I'm a fan of rebounding, as you can tell from chapter 10, and you might also consider walking, swimming, bicycling, weight training or using a cross-trainer like an elliptical machine, or other exercise that will help you sweat out excess acids from your body. Whatever you choose, do it at least five times a week for at least fifteen minutes (and for up to an hour)—and make sure you sweat. Also, add strength training to your aerobic activity three times a week (on alternate days). Follow the program outlined in chapter 10.

Here again, a written plan will help you zero in on what your body needs—and commit to doing it. Start by writing down your favorite physical activities—get at least five. Put a check by the ones that move your muscles in ways that help your lymphatic system and get you to sweat. Of those, circle the ones you are going to make (or keep as) a regular part of your life. Stick to one you are passionate about, or mix it up if you like variety. Finally, on the chart below, or, better still, on your regular calendar, mark out for at least the next thirty days exactly when and where and with whom you will be doing those things—make appointments with yourself for at least five times a week for at least fifteen minutes (or until you break a sweat).

My Five Favorite Physical Activities   **Good for Lymph/Sweat?**

1. _____   _____
2. _____   _____
3. _____   _____
4. _____   _____
5. _____   _____

Sunday	Monday	Tuesday	Wednesday	Thursday	Friday	Saturday

As with any new exercise program, you should check with your doctor before beginning.

STEP 4. TAKE YOUR SUPPLEMENTS

Once you've got what you drink and eat on track, the next phase is to add the electron-rich supplements described in chapter 9.

I recommend working up to your full doses gradually. Start with one capsule once a day and work up to the full recommended dose. As for the green drink, start by adding just one-quarter of a teaspoon to each liter of water, building up over time to reach the full teaspoon per liter. If you are highly acidic to begin with, try alternating green drink with plain good alkaline water with pH drops initially, and work up to all of your liters containing green powder.

Take capsule supplements with food or drink at least six times a day and liquid colloidal supplements under the tongue and *before* food or drink.

Cindy

I was working excessive hours for an IT start-up that caused me to gain 90 pounds over a three-year period. I then spent almost two years of my time and lots of money trying to lose the weight with doctors, Weight Watchers, professional trainers, extensive exercise, and more—without success. My energy level was extremely low, my hormones were a mess, and I didn't feel on top of my game mentally. That's when I learned about the pH Miracle for healthy weight loss. I was in the third week of the program before I started losing any weight, but then I lost about 25 to 30 pounds within the first twelve weeks. In five months, I lost 70 pounds, eating alkaline and using the recommended supplements. But I didn't exercise. The weight came off naturally! Now I have my health, my hormones are back on track, I have great energy and mental clarity—and people tell me I look ten years younger. This whole experience has evolved my life on many levels, far beyond weight loss.

STEP 5. PREPARE YOUR EMOTIONAL ENVIRONMENT

You now have in place the major components of taking care of your physical body, but your journey isn't complete unless you also take care of your mind, heart, and soul, as discussed in chapter 7. You must break the cycle of negative thoughts, emotions, and actions that acidify your body as surely as sugar does. Your whole lifestyle needs to be alkalizing, not just your food and exercise but also your relationships, spirituality, and emotional life. Cleanse yourself emotionally, nourish your spirit, reconnect to your true self. All of you, not just your physical body, needs to transition.

Take stock of where you are mentally, emotionally, and spiritually. Like anything else you seriously mean to accomplish, you must

Mike

I didn't start this plan to lose weight. I am a drummer, and a bad case of tennis elbow as well as pain in my foot and knee were threatening to put an end to that after forty years. The mere thought of losing the ability to play motivated me to action. I was

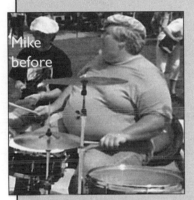

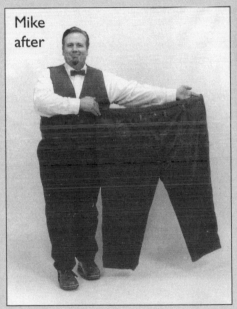

very fat, however: 435 pounds. Losing weight was not my specific goal; it was just what my body decided to do once it got healthy and alkaline. I lost 100 pounds in the first 100 days. I also lost an entire foot off my waistline! I experienced a whole new level of energy within seventy-two

© The Picture People

hours on the program, and after two weeks my elbow and knee pain were completely gone. I felt more like nineteen than forty-nine!

Then, I kept right on losing. I kept having to pull my belt tighter and tighter, and still my pants were sagging off me. After another four months, I was down another 85 pounds. Now I weigh just 235 pounds. I'm nearly half the man I used to be! And I don't plan on stopping anytime soon. I want to see just how far I can go toward being the healthiest I can be. Two things I know for sure: (1) I still need to lose some weight and (2) this is the plan that will allow me to do it. What I am doing *works*.

I'm awed myself by this tremendous success. I don't even feel like I need to have any willpower to make it happen. I always ate a lot, and nothing much has changed in that regard. I just eat the *right* food, alkaline food. I try to eat lots of green food, and most of it raw: avocados, broccoli, peppers, celery, lettuce, spinach. I eliminated meat, eggs, dairy, and (for the most part) processed sugars from my diet. I still eat some crackers, but no bread. The only hard one to let go of has been spaghetti.

I drink 5 to 7 liters of green drink every day. When I'm done with one liter, I just fill up another. I don't drink anything else except green drink! And I use the sprouted soy powder as well as the clay.

After the first few months I also started an exercise program. [Through that first 100 pounds, all I was doing was my (pretty demanding) new factory job, which I started at the same time as the program.] I walked a mile this morning up and down hills, then came home and jumped ten minutes on my rebounder, then picked up the limbs and sticks on my lawn.

I've created my own strategy for keeping myself accountable for my health and weight. I save my grocery store receipts and post them where everyone can see them. What I buy is what I consume. So I am very aware when picking something up and placing it into the cart that it will show up on the receipt. Some of the things on those receipts I am not especially proud of buying. But it is the truth, and I believe "the truth will set us free"! I stay focused on the fact that I am in charge of this process.

I make sure to keep my stress levels as low as possible and make my spiritual life a priority. I try to tell my family of my love for them in every communication. I've taken personal development seminars to help me on my way to defining and keeping my commitment to self-fulfillment, living without fear, and embracing life's possibilities.

As a result of all this I have greater self-confidence, mental clarity, physical coordination, and stamina. My health has never been better in all my life. And I am still losing weight and feeling full of energy.

make a plan for how you are going to progress in this area, including specific goals and a time frame and schedule. The strategies laid out in chapter 7 will guide you. It's somewhat harder to give you specific recommendations for creating an "action plan" for this step than it is for the others, because we all need our own paths. This is definitely not a one-size-fits-all proposition.

In general, the best way I know to move toward knowing your full, spiritual, self is through daily prayer or meditation. Find a place of peace and quiet, even if that place is only in your own mind, where you can listen for the voice of what people all over the world, throughout history, have called by many names (self, soul, spirit, Brahman, Buddha, Nature, Atman, Christ Consciousness). It is here you will receive renewed physical, mental, and emotional strength for a life lived with love and joy.

You'll also need to enlist your best emotional and psychological self to succeed in this program. It's not a complicated program, but anything so different from what those around you are doing isn't always going to be easy. So show up with your best self, in every aspect. And then use some simple tools to your benefit. Start with setting goals, and keeping tabs on your progress. Commit to your plan. Hold yourself accountable.

STEP 6. SET GOALS AND WRITE THEM DOWN

The best way to make sure you get where you're going on any journey is to know where you are in relation to where you want to be. Set a goal for how much weight you would like to lose (or what weight you would ideally be), or what size waist you want to have on your pants, or what dress size you want to wear. The best gauge of results I know is body mass index (BMI) (see chapter 7). The following charts will help you make a map for yourself, and you can track your progress across it. Don't fall into an obsession with the scale—that never helps—and anyway, the way you feel is the gold standard measurement for how this program is working anyway. Stick to taking your measurements once a week, and note them here as you go along. Pick a regular time to do it, like Sunday evenings, or Saturday mornings, whenever is convenient for you. You should always check your weight and measure your waist, buttocks, hips, thighs, chest, arms, and neck as well.

My Measurements					
	Start	Week 1	Week 2	Week 3	Week 4
Date					
Weight (pounds)					
Waist (inches)					
Buttocks					
Hips					
Thighs					
Chest					
Upper arms					
Neck					

	Week 5	Week 6	Week 7	Week 8
Date				
Weight (pounds)				
Waist (inches)				
Buttocks				
Hips				
Thighs				
Chest				
Upper arms				
Neck				

	Week 9	Week 10	Week 11	Week 12
Date				
Weight (pounds)				
Waist (inches)				
Buttocks				
Hips				
Thighs				
Chest				
Upper arms				
Neck				

I also recommend getting your blood pressure, blood cholesterol, blood pH, blood glucose, urine pH, saliva pH, and body fat percentage checked just before you begin, then again after twelve weeks. If you check any of these more regularly, or if there are any other markers, like blood sugar or heart rate, that you normally track, keep a log of all your results in your daily log, as described below.

	Before	After
Blood pressure		
Cholesterol		
pH of blood		
pH of morning urine		
pH of morning saliva		
Blood glucose		
Body fat		

Keep a daily log or journal of your experiences on the pH Miracle Living program. That will help you track what works best for you, and what you need to work on, and see if there is anyplace you need to modify your approach. It helps you keep your commitment to yourself—and see, in black and white, how it pays off, both tangibly (lost pounds and inches) and intangibly (found energy and elevated mood). A sample entry follows; a blank appears in the appendix (page 350) for you to copy and fill out.

DAILY JOURNAL

Date: January 1

Hours slept: 7

Overall energy levels: not so high, and it dipped around 3 P.M.

Overall mood: so-so; I had a spat with my boss

Daily health markers (optional): blood glucose 110 at 8 A.M. and 95 at 11 P.M.; resting heart rate: 85

Exercise: Dancing to music
Duration: 20 minutes

Alkaline Water: _____ liters
How many liters were green drink (with green powder and pH drops)? _____
How many liters had soy sprouts? _____

Supplements:
Omega-3s and omega-6s: 1 (500 mg) capsule 6 times a day with food or green drink
L-carnitine: 1 (200 mg) capsule 6 times a day with food or green drink
Garcinia cambogia or HCA/chromium/tyrosine: 1 combination 500 mg capsule 6 times a day with food or green drink
Clay: Mix 1 teaspoon in 2 to 4 ounces of warm water and drink at least 6 times a day
Other: Lower bowel cleanser 4 (500 mg) capsules every 4 hours

Food: (a typical day not on the cleanse)
7 A.M.: 1 liter of green drink with supplements
8 A.M.: AvoRado Kid Super Green Shake (page 221)
9 A.M.: 1 liter of green drink with supplements
10:30 A.M.: bowl of Green Gazpacho (page 239)
Noon: 1 liter of green drink with supplement
1 P.M.: Large green salad with small piece of wild tuna
2:30 P.M.: 1 liter of green drink with supplements
4 P.M.: Handful of soaked almonds
5 P.M.: 1 liter of green drink with supplements
6 P.M.: Medley of steamed veggies including broccoli, celery, and cucumbers, with olive oil and steamed buckwheat
7:30 P.M.: 1 liter of green drink with supplements

Emotions:
Notable feelings. Include any connection to what you ate/drank/took:
Fight with boss. Drinking green drink helped me calm down afterward.

STEP 7. CLEANSE YOUR BODY FROM THE INSIDE OUT

Okay, *now* you're ready to start the clock running on your twelve weeks. Consider this "last" step as, actually, the beginning of the cycle. The true pH Miracle for weight loss begins with a two- or three-week "cleanse," or "liquid feast," which I'll describe here. For that time, your food and supplement choices will be somewhat different from what's already been described, although your hydration, exercise, and emotional work stay constant. Once you're done with your feast (so called because it is so much more than a fast), you'll move back to the alkaline eating plan you've already been working toward, like the one described in chapter 8. (See chapter 12 for menu plans to guide and inspire you.)

A liquid feast is like a bit of internal spring cleaning. It allows you the same kind of renewal. It allows you to move out a lot of acids and toxins that have built up over months and years of non-alkaline living. An acidic body doesn't properly digest food, and a cleanse helps you clear out all the undigested food and acids from your gastrointestinal system.

Here's what you do: Eat as much as you want, as often as you want, as long as all your food is green, electron-rich, and pureed or juiced. Be sure to include good fats, like avocados, and olive, flax, and fish oils. You must avoid all acidic foods entirely for the duration of the liquid feast. As usual, as much as possible of what you eat or drink should be raw. Not only will this infusion of alkaline energy rid your body of accumulated toxins and acids, but also it will allow your body to devote all of the energy it would otherwise need for digestion to healing you—from the inside out.

As the acids work their way out of your body, you may experience symptoms of detoxification, including bad breath, muscle aches, rashes, congestion, and allergy- or cold-like symptoms. If so: congratulations! The cleanse is working. I call this a "healing crisis." But only a small percentage of people experience these symptoms, and they are generally remedied by full hydration. If you've worked gradually through the initial steps in this program, you're less likely to encounter symptoms now. In order to let your body do the work it needs to during this time, I recommend as much rest and relaxation for you as possible. You can do low-impact exercise (like rebounding!), but if you are tired you need to rest to allow your body to cleanse and regenerate.

On the plus side, most of my clients drop 10 to 20 pounds during this first phase, as toxic acids and wastes leave the body, along with the fat that was holding them.

In addition, a word of warning: Stake out the closest bathrooms at home, work, and play, because you will be visiting often. Most acid-bound fat will come out through the bowels and the urinary tract. It can also come out through the skin or mouth, accounting for the rashes and bad breath side effects, or even the vagina. It's all good. Getting acids out of your body is always for the best, no matter what the route or the short-term discomfort. There are worse things than pee-ing your way to health!

If you need to lose 50 pounds or less, you should do the liquid feast for the first fourteen days of your twelve-week program. If you're shedding more, stay on it for twenty-one days. You'll find menu plans for ten days on the cleanse below; just start again at day 1 to continue, or repeat the days you liked best. For the first day I'll give you the full schedule, including supplements, exercise, and drinks. After that, the menu plans basically rotate out which recipes you follow each day to make sure you enjoy some variety in your program. The rest of the schedule remains the same every day.

Consider this a guideline. You may have to adjust the times to fit your own daily schedule. Take all supplements as directed here, or follow the directions on their individual bottles.

Day 1

7 A.M. **(or, upon waking)**	Drink 1 liter of green drink (water with pH drops and powdered greens), with fresh lemon juice if desired. Optional: add 1 teaspoon of soy sprouts powder, or eat the soy just before you drink the green drink.
7:30 A.M.	Take 5 drops of colloidal chromium under your tongue; or take chromium capsules at 8 A.M. as directed.

7:35 A.M.	Exercise for 15 minutes, preferably on a rebounder.
8 A.M.	Drink Minty Mock Malt (page 227). With your shake, take 1 (1000 mg) omega-3 capsule, 1 teaspoon of powdered soy sprouts, and 1 teaspoon of cold-pressed flaxseed oil (which you can mix into your shake).
	Take a mild herbal laxative (see Box), 4 (500 mg) capsules.
	Take 1 teaspoon of clay stirred into 4 ounces of warm water.
	Take 1 (200 mg) capsule of carnitine, 1 (500 mg) capsule of Garcinia cambogia, 1 (200 mg) capsule of L-tyrosine and (if you haven't taken the colloidal liquid form already) 1 (200 mg) capsule chromium.

HERBAL LAXATIVES

You'll have an array of choices at your local natural food store of mild herbal laxatives. The precise combination you get isn't important, as long as you choose something natural and gentle, formulated around one or more bowel-cleansing herbs such as Cascara Sagrada, psyllium seed, butternut root bark, rhubarb root, and licorice root.

9 A.M.–12 noon	Drink 2 to 3 liters of green drink with the optional soy sprouts powder.
Noon	Take 4 (500 mg) capsules of mild herbal laxative with last of morning green drink.
12:30 P.M.	Same as 7:30 A.M.
1 P.M.	Drink Esther's Garden Soup (page 235) and take the same supplements as listed at 8 A.M.
2–5 P.M.	Drink 1 to 2 liters of green drink with the optional soy sprouts powder.

4 P.M.	Take 4 (500 mg) capsules of mild herbal laxative with some green drink.
5:30 P.M.	Same as 7:30 A.M.
6:00 P.M.	Eat Spicy Tomato Cabbage Soup (page 247) and take the same supplements as listed at 8 A.M., except the laxative.
7–9 P.M.	Drink 1 liter of green drink or plain water with pH drops and lemon juice.
8 P.M.	Take 4 (500 mg) capsules of mild herbal laxative with some green drink or water.

Day 2

Breakfast	Mock Muesli (without the almonds) (page 242)
Lunch	Madrid Gazpacho (page 242)
Dinner	Roasted Red Pepper and Fennel Bisque (without the tofu) (page 246)

Day 3

Breakfast	AvoRado Kid Super Green Shake (page 221)
Lunch	GRASSOUP (page 238)
Dinner	Creamy Cauliflower Confetti Soup (page 234)

Day 4

Breakfast	Carol's Creamy Veggie Soup (page 230)
Lunch	Soothing Cooling Tomato Soup (page 246)
Dinner	Rich Creamy Onion Soup (use fresh almond milk instead of coconut cream) (page 244)

Day 5

Breakfast	AvoRadoColada Shake (page 223)
Lunch	TVP (Tomato, Vegetable, Pesto) Soup (leave out potato) (page 249)
Dinner	Montana Asparagus Soup (page 243)

Day 6

Breakfast	Lemon Ginger Broth (add veggies if you want to) (page 241)

Lunch   Avocado Mint Soup (page 229)
Dinner   Fresh Tomato Basil Soup (page 237)

Day 7
Breakfast Celery/Cauliflower Soup (you can use broccoli instead of cauliflower) (page 230)
Lunch   Grapefruit/Avocado Salsa (pureed) (page 282) (you can use tomatoes instead of grapefruit)
Dinner   Vegetable Minestrone (page 250)

Day 8
Breakfast Lemon Lime Shake (page 226)
Lunch   French Gourmet Puree (page 236)
Dinner   Fresh vegetable juice (any combo of greens juiced; spinach, celery, parsley, kale, cucumber, etc.)

Day 9
Breakfast Cream of Broccoli Soup (use fresh almond milk or coconut water in place of coconut cream) (page 233)
Lunch   Green Gazpacho (page 239)
Dinner   Cream of Zucchini Soup (page 233)

Day 10
Breakfast Cream of Asparagus Soup (use fresh almond milk or fresh coconut water blended with the fresh meat of a Thai coconut instead of coconut cream) (page 232)
Lunch   AvoRado Kid Super Green Shake (page 221)
Dinner   Veggie Almond Chowder (page 250)

You may substitute any recipe suitable for the cleanse from the recipes in chapter 12, or from *The pH Miracle* or *The pH Miracle for Diabetes*—either recipes listed as part of the cleanse plans in any of the books, or any drink, shake, or soup that's entirely green and alkaline—and pureed. The suggested menu plans give you an idea of the combinations you might consider, but please, use the recipes you like best! Whatever you choose, liquefy all soups or shakes in your blender or food processor.

Always eat/drink until you are satisfied but not too full. If at any time of day you feel hungry, you can have more soup, shake, or green drink. Or you can make and drink fresh vegetable juice (using mainly green vegetables and definitely avoiding carrot or beet during the Feast because of their sugar content). Check the recipe chapter and our previous books for suggested juicing combinations. For maximum alkalizing benefits, mix one part vegetable juice with ten parts of electron rich alkaline water, and add 5 pH drops.

After your fourteen or twenty-one days are through, you need to ease your body back into the normal digestive process. Keep the first meal of the day a soup, shake, or green drink for a while. Add in co-conut and avocado to your soups and shakes. For other meals, move first to chunkier soups —the same ones you've been using, but not pureed. Once your body's adjusted to that, move on to salads, then slowly start adding in the 20 to 30 percent foods, the less alkaline and cooked foods, that cover the smaller portion of your plate at each meal.

As you enter this second phase, the amount of acids your body is throwing off lessens—much of what needed to go has already gone. New, healthy tissue is being formed on the strength of the true nu-trition you are providing your body with. You'll feel renewed strength and rejuvenation. You'll enter the third phase sometime after completing the full twelve-week program when you have reached your ideal permanent weight and are in your most healthy state physically, emotionally, and spiritually.

The hardest part of the Liquid Feast—and, in fact, of this whole program—is deciding to begin. Once you've started down the path, you'll begin experiencing the healthy, energetic, strong—and lean!—body you are meant to live in, and you'll never want to turn back.

Chapter 12

Let's Eat

Come forth into the light of things. Let nature be your teacher.
—WORDSWORTH

As fascinating as the science might be behind all this, when it comes right down to it what really matters is *What am I going to eat?* This is where Shelley comes in. Her incredible creativity in the kitchen makes this program pleasurable, as you will discover for yourself as soon as you start trying the recipes in this chapter. We hope you will find the art of cooking this way. Experiment. Modify. Most of all, enjoy!

A handful of the recipes included here have appeared in our previous books. We felt some of the basic recipes we used most often would be important to have immediately on hand as you begin this program. You can of course find more recipes in those books when you are ready to branch out; there are also recipes available on our website (www.pHmiracleliving.com).

To get you started on this exciting new journey, Shelley's giving you here fourteen days' worth of suggested menus to begin after your cleanse is finished. There's nothing magic about these combinations; you can trade meals depending on what you have on hand or what you are in the mood for. You can always substitute any meal with a big salad. These menus are just meant to make it easier for you to eat this way as you begin. Consider these menus as suggestions, not requirements. The recipes for all the dishes mentioned follow. As long as you eat alkaline, and eat until you are satisfied, not stuffed, you'll get the results you are after.

Day 1
    Breakfast AvoRado Kid Super Green Shake (page 221)
    Lunch Cabbage Delight (page 254) with Spelt Flour Tortillas (page 310)
    Dinner Stir-Fry UN-Cashew Chicken (page 316) with steamed quinoa or buckwheat
               Mixed greens salad with dressing of choice

Day 2
    Breakfast Minty Mock Malt (page 227)
    Lunch Dream Castle Salad (page 256)
               Lemon and Tomato Dressing (page 275)
    Dinner Spelt/Quinoa Manicotti Shells with Marinara Sauce (page 310)
               Mixed greens salad with dressing of choice

Day 3
    Breakfast 2–3 Seed Pancakes with Whipped Topping (page 304)
               Roasted Leek Ginger Soup (page 245)
    Lunch Large Mung Bean Sprout and Avocado Salad (page 258)
    Dinner Artichokes Stuffed with Pesto (page 288)
               Esther's Hearty Sprouted Lentil Burgers (page 296)
               Raw spinach salad with dressing of choice

Day 4
    Breakfast Roasted Red Pepper and Fennel Bisque (page 246)
               Dill Toasties (page 330)
    Lunch Crispy Oriental Salad with dressing (page 255)
               Baked Tofu (page 292)

Dinner   Steamed Fish and Greens in Coconut Water (page
               315)
               Mixed greens salad, cherry tomatoes, and dressing of
               choice

Day 5
Breakfast Michael's Bars (page 331) with fresh Almond Rose
               Milk (page 221)
Lunch   Baked Eggplant Slices (page 291) with large mixed
               green salad
               K&L Thousand Island Dressing (page 274)
Dinner   Tofu Sausage (from Mexican Stack Up) (page 299)
               Pepper and onion salad with Casper's Ranch Dress-
               ing (page 267)

Day 6
Breakfast Zucchini Salad (page 266)
Lunch   Stacks (of your choice) (page 314)
Dinner   Mixed Veggie Lentils (page 300)
               Greens salad with Garlic French Dressing (page 270)

Day 7
Breakfast Avocado Margarita (page 290)
               Steamed raw buckwheat
Lunch   Large mixed green salad with Esther's All-Purpose
               Dressing (page 269)
Dinner   Spaghetti Squash with Pumpkin Seed Pesto (page
               309)
               Steamed broccoli with oil and lemon
               Avocado and Tomato slices

Day 8
Breakfast Lemon Ginger Broth (page 241)
               Tera's Hearty Party (page 264)
Lunch   Tofu Potato Salad/Stuffed in Tomato Blossom (page
               265)
               Mixed greens with K&L Ranch Dressing (page 273)

Dinner   Cream of Broccoli Soup (page 233)
Salad with dressing of choice
Sprouted Lentil Crackers (page 338)

Day 9
Breakfast Mock Muesli (page 338)
Lunch   Assorted raw veggie sticks, soaked almonds
Spicy Southwestern Chipotle Sauce (page 284)
Lavender Mint Tea (page 225)
Dinner   Coconut Cream Fish Fillet (page 293)
Salad with dressing of choice
Steamed quinoa

Day 10
Breakfast Avocado Mint Soup (page 229)
Lunch   Barbeque Buffalo Chips (page 325)
Salad with Lemon Basil Dressing (page 275)
Dinner   Lettuce/Cabbage Wraps with Hot, Sweet Sauce (page 298)
Sandy's Almond Joy (2) (page 336)

Day 11
Breakfast Cream of Asparagus Soup (page 232)
Savory Alkalarian Crackers (page 337)
Lunch   Brussels Sprouts Sauté (page 292)
Deliciously Scrumptious Happy Salmon Burgers (page 294)
Dinner   Roasted Cajun Vegetables (page 203)
TVP Soup (page 249)
Greens salad with dressing of choice
Michael's Bars (2) (page 331)

Day 12
Breakfast Almost Apple Pie (page 324)
Lunch   Michael's Pizza Tortilla (page 300)
Dinner   Garlic Cauliflower "Potatoes" (page 298)
Spicy Coconut Crusted Salmon (page 313)

Roasted Garlic and Sun-Dried Tomato Cream Sauce (page 314)

Salad with Esther's All-Purpose Dressing (page 269)

Day 13

Breakfast   AvoRadoColada Shake (page 223)

Lunch   Fresh Tomato Basil Soup (page 237)

Mixed greens with K&L Thousand Island Dressing (page 274)

Dinner   Purple Edamame Stir-Fry (page 301)

Salad with Sesame Soy (Braggs) Dressing (page 280)

Day 14

Breakfast   Lemon Lime Shake (page 226)

Lunch   Large mixed greens salad with Southwest Caesar Dressing (page 278)

Spelt Flour Tortillas (page 310)

Dinner   Esther's Garden Soup (page 235)

Raw Slim Sticks (page 334)

RECIPE INDEX

ENTRÉES/SIDE DISHES

DRINKS AND SHAKES

Almond Rose Milk

Contributed by Shawnda Hansen

MAKES 20–24 OZ

1 cup raw almonds
3¼ cups pure water
¼–½ cup rose water (Carlo brand)
¼ tsp. stevia powder
3 dashes nutmeg

Soak almonds in 2 cups of the pure water overnight in the refrigerator. In blender, pulse-chop, then blend almonds and water. Slowly add the remaining pure water and rose water. Add stevia, blend until smooth. Use cheesecloth or panty hose to strain almond pulp from milk. Pour into glasses and add a dash of nutmeg to garnish.

AvoRado Kid Super Green Shake or Pops

SERVES 1

This is by far our favorite cool green shake. It's a great way to get the concentrated nutrition of green powder and soy sprouts powder, and the added benefits of God's great butter, avocado. The cucumber and lime act as a coolant to the body and the essential fats in the avocado and soy sprouts give the energy elements to make this shake one that you can burn on for many hours. We have enjoyed this shake for breakfast, lunch, dinner, or as a great anytime snack, as well as on the cleanse. This is a fantastic way to get these nutrients in your kids. In the summer, try the pops for a cool frozen treat.

1 avocado

½ English cucumber (organic and usually wrapped in plastic, if possible)

1 tomatillo

1 lime (peeled)

2 cups fresh spinach

2 scoops soy sprouts powder

1 scoop of green powder

1 pkg. stevia

6–8 ice cubes

Place all ingredients in a blender (I prefer Vita-Mix with the plunger) on high speed and blend to a thick smooth consistency. Serve immediately.

For Pops: Pour into ice cube trays, frozen pop trays, or small paper cups and freeze. Thaw the cups a little and remove the frozen shake and chop up and enjoy as a slush, if so desired.

Variations:
- Add 1 tsp. almond butter for a nuttier flavor.
- Add coconut milk or Fresh Silky Almond Milk (page 223) for a creamier shake.
- Make a parfait by layering the shake with layers of dehydrated unsweetened coconut and sprinkle some of the coconut on top.
- Substitute a grapefruit or a lemon for the lime for a different taste.
- Add 1 Tbs. fresh grated ginger
- Use some of the new Frontier flavorings that are bottled in oil (without alcohol) for a new exciting twist of flavor.

AvoRadoColada Shake

SERVES 1

This refreshing shake has additional lycopene found in ruby-red grape-fruits. The blending of the meat and water of a young (Thai) coconut will give it a tropical essence. Enjoy! This is one of the all-time favorite shakes served at our pH Miracle retreats.

½ English cucumber (if organic do not peel or seed)
Juice from ½ large ruby red grapefruit
The meat and water of one young Thai coconut
1 avocado
1 cup fresh organic spinach (optional)
1 scoop (tsp.) greens powder
1 scoop (tsp.) soy sprouts powder
1 tsp. raw green stevia powder (Frontier brand) or stevia to taste
½ tsp. vanilla flavoring (Frontier brand)
½ tsp. coconut flavoring (Frontier brand)
8–10 ice cubes

Place cucumber, grapefruit juice, coconut meat, and coconut water in blender and blend. Then place all remaining ingredients in blender with ice last and blend quickly until thick and creamy. Serve immediately.

Variation:
- Sprinkle freeze-dried dehydrated coconut flakes on top or layer in parfait glass with shake and coconut flakes alternating.

Fresh Silky Almond Milk

SERVES 4–6

4 cups of fresh raw almonds
Pure water
White knee-high nylon stocking (for straining)

Soak the raw almonds overnight in a bowl of water. In the morning drain the almonds and fill blender with the almonds about a third full (2 cups), then add pure water to fill the blender up. Blend on high speed until you have a white creamy-looking milk. Take a nylon stocking (I use a washed white knee-high nylon stocking) and pour the mixture through it over a bowl or pan, and let it drain. Squeeze with your hand to get the last of the milk through the nylon. (The meal and skins left in the stocking can be used in the shower for a great body scrub.)

You will have approximately 1 quart of silky raw beautiful almond milk left ready to use for soups, shakes, or puddings. Thin to desired consistency with water. Almond milk will keep fresh for about 3 days in the refrigerator. You can also drink this plain or add a bit of stevia for sweeter almond milk.

George's Breakfast Pizzazz

Contributed by Mary Jo and George Walter

SERVES 1

½ blender jar mixed baby greens (and sprouts)
½–1 cucumber
2 garlic cloves
2-inch–6-inch pieces of thin rhubarb
¼ tsp. Braggs Liquid Aminos
½ cup onion, Vidalia preferred
2 oz. extra-virgin olive oil
½ cup distilled water
¼ tsp. dried mustard powder
¼ tsp. dried oregano
Few celery seeds
RealSalt and white pepper to taste
Pinch cayenne pepper

In blender, on low speed to start, blend all ingredients. Increase speed and blend until smooth.

Hint: Rhubarb is a great substitute for tomatillos in shakes. Mix can easily be doubled.

Lavender Mint Tea

Contributed by Lisa El-Kerdi
Best in Show, pH Miracle 2004 Recipe Contest

SERVES 8

1½ cups fresh mint leaves
½ cup fresh lavender flowers
8–10 cups pure boiling water
Stevia to taste (optional)

In large saucepan, place mint and lavender. Add boiling water, cover, and steep on low for 5 to 10 minutes, to desired strength. Strain. Add stevia if desired and more boiling water if too strong. May be served hot or cold.

Infusions: Prepare this tea as a flavoring for sparkling mineral water by decreasing the amount of water used to 2 cups. Prepare as directed, strain, and cool. When ready to serve, pour chilled mineral water into glasses, add infusion to taste, and enjoy!

Lemon Ginger Tea

Contributed by Lisa El-Kerdi

SERVES 1

1 thumb-size piece of fresh gingerroot, peeled
1 cinnamon stick
Rind of ½ lemon
8 cups pure boiling water
Juice of 1–2 lemons
Stevia to taste (optional)

Place ginger, cinnamon stick, and lemon rind in saucepan. Pour boiling water over spices and steep on low heat for 10 to 15 minutes. Add lemon juice and stevia (if desired) before serving. Discard spices and serve, adding more boiling water if too strong.

Variation:
• For a winter spice tea, add ½ tsp. cloves and the rind of ½ orange.

Lemon Lime Shake

Contributed by Donna Downing

SERVES 1

1 avocado, peeled and seeded
½ English cucumber
1 lime, peeled
2 lemons, juiced
1 young coconut, juice and meat
1 packet stevia
8 oz. ice cubes

In Vita-Mix, layer ingredients in order listed. Blend on low to start. As liquid incorporates, increase speed to high and blend until smooth and frothy. Add more ice for sorbet-type consistency. Serve immediately.

Variation:
- Add 1 tsp. greens powder and 2 tsps. soy sprouts powder to increase nutrition in shake.

Minty Mock Malt

Contributed by Matthew and Ashley Rose Lisonbee

SERVES 2

½ **English cucumber**
1 **lime, juiced**
1 **grapefruit, juiced**
1 **avocado**
1 **cup raw spinach**
½ **can of coconut milk**
1 **scoop (1 tsp.) SuperGreens powder (Innerlight Foundation brand)**
2 **scoops (2 tsps.) soy sprouts powder**
8–10 **drops Prime pH drops**
2–4 **sprigs fresh mint leaves or use ½ tsp. mint flavoring—no alcohol (Frontier brand)**
14 **ice cubes**

Combine all ingredients into a Vita-Mix or any other blender and blend to desired consistency.

Tip: Use ice cubes for refreshing morning malt or use no ice cubes for making your kids great tasty Popsicles.

Soda Shoppe Shakes

Contributed by Lisa El-Kerdi
Best in Show, pH Miracle 2004 Recipe Contest

MAKES 2 LARGE OR 4 SMALL

2 young white coconuts

At least 3 hours before serving, open and blend flesh and water of 1 coconut in blender or Vita-Mix. If coconut has a lot of water and little flesh, add coconut oil and flakes to thicken. Freeze in ice cube tray or 6 oz. plastic cups. May be prepared and frozen several days in advance. At time of final preparation or up to several hours prior, open and blend second coconut. At this time add desired flavorings (see Variations). Add stevia to taste if necessary. Refrigerate until serving time. Remove frozen coconut mixture from freezer. If using plastic cups, stand in pot of warm water for a minute to loosen. Add to unfrozen mixture and blend until creamy. Add ice cubes if necessary. Pour into glasses, add straw, enjoy!

The following are optional additions and may be used to create different flavors and textures. Measurements are general and may be altered to taste.

½–1 tsp. alcohol-free vanilla extract
½ tsp. alcohol-free almond extract
1 Tbs. carob powder
Stevia to taste, if desired
1 tsp.–1 Tbs. coconut oil
Unsweetened dried coconut flakes to taste
Ice cubes to thicken (optional)

Variations:
- Coconut Shake: Simply blend coconuts as desired. For more intense coconut flavor or thicker shake, add coconut oil and flakes.

- Creamy Vanilla Shake: Add vanilla to taste.
- Fudgy Carob Shake: Add vanilla, almond, and carob.

SOUPS

Avocado Mint Soup

Contributed by Ashley Lisonbee

SERVES 6

**3 Tbs. grapeseed or olive oil
6 green onions, sliced
1 garlic clove, crushed
4 Tbs. spelt flour
2½ cups vegetable broth
2–3 tsps. lemon juice
½ tsp. grated lemon zest
⅔ cup coconut milk
⅔ cup coconut cream
1½ mint, chopped
RealSalt and pepper, to taste
2 avocados, sliced into cubes
1 cup spinach, minced
Mint sprigs for garnish**

In a soup pot, heat grapeseed or olive oil. Add green onions, garlic, and spelt flour. Simmer. Stir in the remaining ingredients, mix well. Add avocados and spinach last, warm-stirring gently. Serve, garnishing with mint sprigs.

Carol's Creamy Veggie Soup

Contributed by Carol Murie

SERVES 4

½ large onion, diced
⅛ cup coconut oil
2 medium carrots, sliced
2 medium zucchini, sliced
2 cups broccoli
1 quart vegetable broth
1 potato, cubed (optional)
½ tsp. celery seed
1 tsp. ground cumin
1 tsp. Celtic Salt
1 tsp. Zip (Spice Hunter)
1 cup almond milk
Fresh sprouts for garnish

Sauté onion in coconut oil until transparent. Add carrots, zucchini, and broccoli. Sauté for 5 minutes until crisp-tender. Add broth, potato, and seasonings. Simmer until veggies are tender (10 minutes or less). Stir in almond milk, heat through. At serving, garnish each bowl with fresh sprouts.

Celery/Cauliflower Soup

SERVES 6–8

1 onion, peeled and chopped
1 Tbs. oil (olive oil or Udo's)
1 bunch celery, trimmed and chopped, save leaves for garnish
1 head cauliflower, trimmed and chopped
1–2 qts. vegetable stock

½–1 qt. almond milk
Salt, pepper, and seasoning of choice to taste

In a large soup pan, steam-fry onion in a little oil for about 5 minutes without browning. In food processor, pulse-chop celery and cauliflower until finely chopped. Add cauliflower and celery mix to pan, warm until tender. Add vegetable stock and almond milk. Simmer for 15 to 30 minutes, or leave raw if desired. Puree the soup mixture in blender, until smooth texture. Season to taste, serve warm or cold.

Chipotle Pepper Soup

Variations: Pumpkin Eater's Soup
Vegetable and Tofu with Chipotle Pepper Sauce

Contributed by Linnette Webster
First place, pH Miracle 2004 Recipe Contest
Transitional Category

Chipolte Pepper imparts a wonderful smoked flavor to this dish.

2 zucchini, chopped in ½-inch cubes
1 tsp. Italian seasonings, if desired
2 Tbs. olive oil
1 onion, chopped
1 celery stalk, chopped
2 garlic cloves, minced
2 carrots, cut in ⅜-inch slices
1 red potato, ½-inch cubes (optional)
½ red bell pepper, ⅝-inch diced
RealSalt to taste

Cube tofu into ⅝-inch squares, salt (or drizzle with Bragg Liquid Aminos). In a skillet on medium-high heat, brown tofu in 1 Tbs.

olive oil. Add water to skillet and mix well. Set aside to use as addition to soup or vegetable dish. Brown zucchini and seasoning in olive oil for 2 minutes. Add to skillet, steam-frying for 2 minutes, onion, celery, garlic. Add to skillet carrots, steam-fry 2 minutes. Add potato, steam-fry for 4 minutes. Add red bell pepper, steam-fry for 2 minutes. Season to taste.

Optional:
1 carton tofu
RealSalt to taste or Bragg Liquid Aminos
1 Tbs. olive oil
1 cup pure water

Cream of Asparagus Soup

Contributed by Ashley Lisonbee

SERVES 4

2 Tbs. olive oil
⅓ yellow onion, chopped
2 garlic cloves, minced
1 bunch of organic asparagus, chopped
3½ cups vegetable broth, organic
6 oz. coconut cream, organic
2 tsps. RealSalt
1½ tsps. Deliciously Dill (Spice Hunter)
½ tsp. fresh lemon peel, grated
2 Tbs. lemon juice (fresh)

In soup pot, heat oil on medium. Add onion, garlic, and asparagus and sauté for 3 or 4 minutes, until veggies are tender. Add veggie broth and warm for 8 to 10 minutes. Reduce heat to low. Stir in coconut cream and seasonings. Warm for 5 more minutes. Serve warm.

Cream of Broccoli Soup

Contributed by Ashley Lisonbee

SERVE 4–6

2 Tbs. olive oil
1 onion, diced
2 cups broccoli
1 Tbs. grapeseed oil
4½ cups vegetable broth
⅔ cup coconut cream
1/16 tsp. paprika plus dash for garnish
Salt and pepper to taste
½ tsp. Herbes de Provence (Spice Hunter)
2½ cups avocado, diced

Chop onion. Peel and chop broccoli stalks into small pieces. In soup pot, heat oil to medium low, gently sauté onion and broccoli for 5 minutes. Add vegetable broth and broccoli florets and let simmer on low for 15 minutes. Remove from heat, letting soup cool. In blender, puree half of the soup mixture. Pour back into soup pot and mix. Gently stir in coconut cream until mixed thoroughly. Add spices and diced avocado. Serve warm, garnishing with a dash of paprika.

Cream of Zucchini Soup

SERVES 2–4

This is a satisfying creamed soup that is great anytime and also while on the cleanse. The Spicy Garlic Herb Bread Seasoning (Spice Hunter) kicks it up a little to make it especially warming *to the body. Experiment with different spices.*

1 large onion, chopped
3 zucchini, sliced in ¼-inch thick slices
3 ripe tomatoes, cut into large chunks
1–2 cups of water
1 avocado
1 tsp. Spicy Garlic Herb Bread Seasoning (Spice Hunter)
2 tsps. RealSalt

Steam-fry onion in a soup pan until softened and almost clear (3 to 5 minutes). Add zucchini and continue to steam-fry until zucchini is bright green and softened a bit (3 to 4 minutes). Add tomatoes and steam-fry 1 to 2 minutes more. Place all the steam-fried ingredients into a blender (I use Vita-Mix), and add the water and avocado. Blend on high until smooth and creamy, and with blender running, sprinkle in the seasoning and salt to taste. Serve immediately.

Creamy Cauliflower Confetti Soup

SERVES 4–6

This soup is deceptively creamy; if you didn't know better, you'd swear it had dairy in it, but it's the combination of Fresh Silky Almond Milk with pureed roasted cauliflower and celery root that does the trick. The roasted veggie bits give it its confetti appearance. Sprinkle roasted bell peppers over the top and a dash of the Zip for more color.

1 head cauliflower
3 yellow crookneck squash
4 zucchini
2 yellow onions
2 pkg. cherry tomatoes
½ celery root
Grapeseed oil
8 cloves garlic
1 qt. Fresh Silky Almond Milk (page 223)
1 container Pacific Veggie Broth

Place bite-sized pieces of veggies on nonstick cookie sheets and rub with a little grapeseed oil. Roast until lightly browned in your broiler, 10 to 15 minutes. While veggies are roasting, make the quart of Fresh Silky Almond Milk in your blender. Place almond milk in soup pan. After veggies are roasted, place the cauliflower, half the onions, and half the celery root pieces in the blender. Add the almond milk and blend together until rich and creamy, then put back into the soup pan. In the food processor, pulse-chop remaining veggies to diced or minced consistency and spoon into the soup. Stir to separate bits. Add 1 container of Pacific brand Veggie Broth and stir well. Enjoy!

Esther's Garden Soup

Contributed by Esther Andreas
Third place, pH Miracle 2004 Recipe Contest
Alkalizing Category

SERVES 4–6

Broth

3 stalks celery
⅛ red onion
1 small garlic clove
¼ cup lemon juice
2 cups warm water
3 Tbs. olive oil
1 tsp. dried sage or 3 Tbs. chopped fresh sage
½ tsp. RealSalt
2 drops stevia

Blend above ingredients until smooth. Pour into large bowl.

Garden Soup Veggies

Use 3 or 4 of the following vegetables to make a colorful soup.

½ cup chopped red pepper
¼ cup jicama, grated
1 small carrot, chopped
1 cup zucchini, grated
½ cup parsnips, grated
½ cup cauliflower, chopped
½ cup broccoli, chopped
1 avocado
Cayenne or ginger for flavor
Fresh parsley, cilantro, green onion, chives for garnish

Add vegetables of choice to soup broth, stir well. Add 1 avocado, cut into bite-sized pieces. Adjust flavors by adding a little cayenne or ginger. Garnish with fresh parsley, fresh cilantro, green onions, or chives.

French Gourmet Puree

Contributed by Eric Prouty
First place, pH Miracle 2004 Recipe Contest
Alkalizing Category

SERVES 6

This is a beautiful soothing alkalizing puree. I often like to double the romaine lettuce juice and thin it out a bit more.

1 avocado
2 stalks celery
1 head romaine lettuce
1 small tomato

1 handful spinach
1 small cucumber, peeled
2 garlic cloves
⅓ onion
Herbes de Provence (Spice Hunter) to taste
2 Tbs. olive oil

Use Green Star/Green Life juicer with plug attachment for purees. Puree all vegetables, feeding onion through last. Mix with Herbes de Provence and olive oil.

Optional: Serve with sprouts sprinkled on top. Enjoy!

Fresh Tomato Basil Soup

Contributed by Ashley Lisonbee

SERVES 4–6

2 lbs. vine-ripe tomatoes
2 tsps. olive oil
1 sweet onion, chopped finely
1 celery stalk, chopped finely
1 carrot, chopped finely
2 garlic cloves, minced
1 tsp. fresh marjoram leaves or ¼ tsp. dried
2 cups water
4–5 Tbs. coconut cream plus extra for garnish
2 Tbs. fresh basil, chopped
RealSalt and fresh ground pepper to taste

Chop tomatoes in half. In food processor, pulse-chop, set aside. In large soup pot, heat olive oil. Add onion, celery, and carrot, and cook over medium-low heat for 4 minutes, stirring occasionally. Add tomatoes, minced garlic, and fresh marjoram. Cook for 2 minutes.

Stir in water and simmer for 15 to 20 minutes until veggies are tender. Remove from heat, letting soup cool slightly. Using food processor, blend soup until smooth. Return soup to pot and heat on low. Add coconut cream and chopped basil. Season with salt and pepper. Ladle soup in bowls. Spoon a small dollop of coconut cream in the center of each serving.

GRASSOUP

SERVES 2–4

This soup is totally raw. I prefer it served cool on a hot day. Garnish with a lemon or lime slice and you could even sip on this as a cooling smoothie by the pool. The fresh dill cut into short little lengths looks like grass shavings floating on the top, hence the name GRASSOUP.

2 English cucumbers, juiced (make in juicer, strain all pulp out)
1 young coconut, water (juice) that is clear, sweet, and very fresh
¾–1 cup Fresh Silky Almond Milk (page 223)
1–2 tsps. fresh dill, cut in short lengths (pressed on the counter with the flat edge of a knife to crush and expose the flavor)

Combine all ingredients in a bowl and stir. Soup should be smooth, creamy, and silky with a beautiful light green color.

Variations:
- Use 2 to 4 tsps. of dehydrated red bell pepper powder (made ahead) to give it an extra sparkling sweet addition.

Dehydrated Red Bell Pepper Powder

Wash, core, seed, and slice several red bell peppers (about ¼-inch thick). Spread on dehydrator sheet and dry completely until snap crisp. Grind to a fine powder in Vita-Mix blender or small coffee grinder. This is a rich, sweet garnishing powder that you can add to soups, salads, wraps, or stir-fry. Store in Tupperware (lasts about 3 months).

Green Gazpacho

Contributed by Eric Prouty
First place, pH Miracle 2004 Recipe Contest
Alkalizing Category

SERVES 4–6

This is a split *recipe that you can prepare simply with no herbs or seasonings, or you can pump it up and make it* robust *with the addition of the herbs. Either way, it's a wonderfully alkalizing soup and very packed with chlorophyll. Our family prefers the robust version.*

Refreshing

2 avocados, cut in chunks
¼ cup fresh lemon juice
3 garlic cloves
6 roma tomatoes, chopped
1 head romaine lettuce, chopped
2 green bell peppers, chopped
1–1½ large English cucumbers (or 2 average size), chopped
½ red onion, chopped

Add all the ingredients to food processor (with S blade) in the following combinations: Mix avocado, lemon juice, and garlic until smooth, empty into bowl. Mix tomatoes and romaine until smooth, empty into bowl. Mix bell peppers, cucumbers, and onion until chunky (approx. ⅛–¼-inch pulse for consistency).

Robust Version

1½ tsps. basil
½ tsp. dill
¼ tsp. oregano
⅛ tsp. sage powder
¼ tsp. RealSalt
2 Tbs. olive oil

Add herbs and salt to oil. Mix well, then add to the gazpacho and enjoy!

Iced Salsa Soup

Contributed by Ashley Lisonbee

SERVES 4

1 Tbs. grapeseed oil
1 orange or red bell pepper, finely chopped
1 green bell pepper, finely chopped
1 sweet onion, finely chopped
3 vine-ripened tomatoes, chopped
1 tsp. chili powder (Spice Hunter)
½ cup water
2 cups vine-ripened tomatoes
RealSalt and pepper to taste
Zip to taste (Spice Hunter)
Fresh cilantro or 3–4 scallions for garnish

In a soup pot, heat grapeseed oil on medium heat. Add the bell peppers and warm, stirring briskly, for 3 minutes. Add onion and cook for 2 more minutes. Add tomatoes and chili powder; continue to warm, stirring frequently for 1 minute. Add water and cover. Turn off heat and let set for 4 or 5 minutes. Transfer soup base to a large bowl. In food processor, puree tomatoes. Stir into soup base. Add seasonings to taste. Refrigerate until cold and serve. Garnish with fresh cilantro or finely chopped scallions.

Lemon Ginger Broth

Contributed by Victoria's Gourmet—Victoria Frerichs
Professional Award, pH Miracle 2004 Recipe Contest

SERVES 4–5

1 can Pacific Organic Vegetable Broth
⅓ can water
4 lemons, zest and juice
4 Tbs. fresh ginger, finely grated
Salt to taste

Combine broth and water. Bring to boil. Add juice and grated zest of lemons. Turn off heat, and let steep like tea. Add ginger. Strain, salt to taste.

Variations:
½ package extra-firm tofu
Cilantro sprigs for garnish

Cut tofu into cubes, lay in bowls. Add hot broth. Garnish top of soup with cilantro sprigs. Serve warm or chilled.

Madrid Gazpacho

Serve 6–8

3 tomatoes
2 cucumbers
1 red bell pepper
1 jalapeño pepper
1 qt. pure water
3 Tbs. olive oil
2 lemons, juiced
1 tsp. cumin
2 tsps. RealSalt
Garlic to taste
Tomato, celery, green onion, cucumber, red bell pepper,
    and avocado for garnish

In food processor, blend all vegetables. Add water, oil, juice, and spices. Blend again in batches if necessary. Serve chilled, garnishing with ¼ cup chopped vegetables of choice.

Mock Muesli

Contributed by Eric Prouty
First place, pH Miracle 2004 Recipe Contest
Alkalizing Category

Serves 1–2

1 avocado
1 cucumber, peeled
1 cup spinach, chopped
3 radishes
10–15 almonds, soaked
½ lime, juiced

Stevia to taste
¼ tsp. cinnamon

Cube avocado and cucumber. In food processor, puree avocado, cucumber, and spinach until smooth. Cut radishes in quarters. Add along with almonds, lime juice, stevia, and cinnamon. Briefly process to desired chunkiness.

Montana Asparagus Soup

Contributed by Michael Steadman
Second place, pH Miracle 2004 Recipe Contest
Transitional Category

SERVES 4

1½ cups filtered water
2 cups asparagus, lightly steamed
⅛ cup asparagus water, warm
½ avocado, peeled and chopped
3 celery stalks, chopped
2 Tbs. Udo's oil
1 tsp. Celtic Salt or RealSalt
2 tsps. lemon juice
1 tsp. lemon pepper (Tones)
4 tsp. onion, minced
1–2 garlic cloves, minced
⅛ tsp. Zip (Spice Hunter)

Blend all ingredients in Vita-Mix until warm.

Variations:
½ avocado, diced
½ cup asparagus, steamed and diced
Herbamare (A. Vogel) and Zip to taste
Spicy Onion Sunflower Seeds (recipe follows) to taste

Spicy Onion Sunflower Seeds

Contributed by Michael Steadman

1 cup sunflower seeds (soaked overnight in purified water)
Bragg Liquid Amino (optional)
RealSalt
Powdered onion
Zip or cayenne pepper

Drain the seeds and place on dehydrator tray screen. Spray with Bragg Liquid amino (optional). Dust with RealSalt, powdered onion, and Zip or cayenne pepper (to taste). Dehydrate for 24 to 36 hours.

Rich Creamy Onion Soup

Contributed by Ashley Lisonbee

SERVES 4

¼ cup olive oil
3 onions, finely chopped
1 garlic clove, crushed
1 tsp. arrowroot powder
2½ cups vegetable broth
2½ cups almond milk
Salt and Zip (Spice Hunter) or crushed red pepper to taste
2–3 tsps. lemon or lime juice
1 bay leaf
1 carrot, finely diced
4 Tbs. coconut cream
2 Tbs. parsley, chopped for garnish

In a soup pan warm the oil, onions, and garlic on low heat for 8 to 10 minutes, stirring frequently. Stir in arrowroot and warm, stirring for 1 minute. Add the vegetable broth, increasing heat to medium, not boiling. Add the almond milk and stir and warm for 5 minutes. Add seasonings, citrus juice, and bay leaf. Cover and simmer on low, 15 minutes. Discard the bay leaf. Stir in carrot and simmer 2 to 3 minutes. Add coconut cream. Add more lemon or lime juice or seasoning to taste. Garnish with parsley. Serve warm and enjoy.

Roasted Leek Ginger Soup

SERVES 4

1 Tbs. olive oil or grapeseed oil
1 leek, cleaned and sliced in ⅓-inch slices
1 tsp. fresh ginger, cut in thin slices
1 cup freshly strained almond milk
2 cups vegetable broth (I use Pacific brand)
½–1 tsp. RealSalt

In a soup pan pour some olive oil or grapeseed oil. Place leek and ginger in oil and stir-fry until softened and browned on edges. Place the leek and ginger in a food processor. Pulse-chop to a diced consistency and place back in soup pan. Add fresh almond milk, veggie broth, and RealSalt. Warm and serve.

Variations:
• Add diced roasted peppers and garlic.

Roasted Red Pepper and Fennel Bisque

Contributed by Lisa El-Kerdi
Best in Show, pH Miracle 2004 Recipe Contest

SERVES 8 (4 OZ.) PORTIONS

4 large red bell peppers
1 small bulb fennel
2 tsps. olive oil
½ cup pure water
1 pkg. soft silken tofu
2 tsps. RealSalt or to taste

Cut peppers in half, seed, and place skin side down on a grill to blacken skins. Cut tops off fennel, reserve for garnish. Rub bulb with olive oil and place on grill. When pepper skins are blackened and fennel is lightly roasted, remove from grill to bowl, taking care not to spill juices. Cover bowl in plastic wrap to steam until cool enough to handle. Thinly slice roasted fennel and place in pot with ½ cup pure water. Simmer gently. Peel peppers, removing all blackened bits and add to pot. Add water just to cover and gently simmer until soft. Blend in batches until smooth, adding tofu to last batch. Combine all and add RealSalt to taste. Serve hot or cold. Snip feathery sprigs of fennel top onto each serving to garnish. Serve with Dill Toasties (page 330).

Soothing Cooling Tomato Soup

SERVES 2

The combination of fresh tomatoes and avocado makes this silky smooth cooling soup high in lycopene and lucene.

6 medium tomatoes, juiced and strained (pour through a fine mesh strainer or a nylon knee-high stocking)

½ avocado
¾ cup fresh coconut water (make sure this is fresh, taken from a
    coconut)
1 cucumber, juiced
RealSalt to taste
Stevia (optional)

Blend all ingredients until smooth. For a sweeter soup, add stevia
to taste.

Spicy Tomato Cabbage Soup

Contributed by Ashley Lisonbee

SERVES 6

1 leek
2 Tbs. grapeseed oil
1 garlic clove, minced
1 tsp. fresh ginger, minced
1 tsp. chili powder
3½ cups vegetable broth
2 cups cabbage, chopped
2 cups organic tomato soup broth
1 cup organic peas
2 Tbs. organic tomato paste
½ tsp. RealSalt
Dash red pepper, crushed (optional)

Wash thoroughly and trim leek, removing ends of leaves, leaving
3 inches of green leaf. Finely slice leek. Combine oil, garlic, leek, and
ginger in a soup pan and warm for 3 or 4 minutes until leek is tender.
Stir chili powder into mixture, mix well. Add veggie broth, increase
heat to medium, stir in cabbage, warm for 5 minutes. Add tomato

soup broth, peas, tomato paste, and salt. Warm another 3 minutes. Add a dash of crushed red pepper for a spicy kick. Serve warm and enjoy!

Swiss Chard Lentil Soup

Contributed by Martha Germany
Honorable Mention, pH Miracle 2004 Recipe Contest

SERVES 4–6

2 cups brown lentils, sprouted
6 cups water
1 bunch Swiss chard, red or green
2–3 garlic cloves, crushed
1 bunch cilantro
1 lemon, juiced or 2 Tbs. to taste
2 tsps. RealSalt
⅓ cup olive oil

Soak lentils overnight and sprout for 2 days. In a soup pot, bring rinsed lentils and the water to a boil. Wash and chop Swiss chard into bit-size pieces. When lentils boil, add chard to top, reduce heat to medium, cover, and simmer for 15 minutes. In a small skillet, steam crushed garlic in a small amount of water. Wash and chop cilantro. Add to garlic and steam until wilted. Add to soup along with lemon juice. Simmer 5 more minutes, add salt to taste. Serve, topping each bowl with 1 or 2 Tbs. olive oil to taste.

Variation:
• Replace 6 cups water suggested with 2 cups vegetable broth and 3 cups water, adjusting more liquid as needed.

TVP Soup (Tomato, Vegetable, Pesto)

Contributed by Carol Murie

SERVES 6–8 (8 OZ.) PORTIONS

⅛–¼ **cup homemade Spring's Pesto (recipe follows)**
4 cups tomatoes, cubed
2 cups green or yellow beans, cut into bite-sized pieces
1 cup asparagus, cut into bite-sized pieces
1 onion, chopped
2 cups broccoli, chopped
1 potato, cubed
4 cups pure water
1 tsp. Celtic Salt
Fresh cilantro, diced cucumbers for garnish

Add all ingredients except garnish to soup pot. Simmer for about 10 minutes, until veggies are slightly soft. To serve, add fresh cilantro and diced cucumbers to garnish.

Time-saver note: Easy to freeze in ice cube trays for quick use in many recipes.

Spring's Pesto

6 garlic cloves
4 cups fresh basil, or 1 cup dried
1 cup fresh parsley
6 Tbs. raw nuts (pine, almond, hazel, pumpkin) or combination
1 cup or more olive oil
1–2 tsp. each salt and pepper
2 Tbs. sun-dried tomatoes

In food processor, pulse-chop, then blend all ingredients into thick paste. Ready for use, plain or in recipes for soup as above. Refrigerate.

Vegetable Minestrone

SERVES 4

2 carrots
2 celery stalks
1 quart vegetable broth
1 cabbage
1 red bell pepper
1 onion
1 zucchini
1 yellow summer squash
Flaxseed oil to taste
Bragg Liquid Aminos to taste
Cayenne pepper to taste

Cut vegetables (preferred). Cover carrots and celery with vegetable broth in soup pot. Cook gently until crisp-tender, add remaining vegetables. Do not overcook. Serve hot with flaxseed oil, Bragg Liquid Aminos, and cayenne to taste.

Veggie Almond Chowder

SERVES 4

3 cups soaked almonds [you can blanch them to remove the skins if desired or make Fresh Silky Almond Milk (page 223) if you don't want the almond meal in your chowder]
1–2 lemons, juiced
1 garlic clove
1 tsp. Garlic Herb Bread Seasoning (Spice Hunter)
1 qt. veggie broth (I use Pacific brand)
2 tsps. dehydrated tomato powder (The Spice House)
1 tsp. RealSalt
½ tsp. celery salt

Black pepper or Zip to taste (Spice Hunter)
¼ tsp. Green Thai curry paste (Thai Kitchen)
1 head broccoli, chopped
1 yellow onion, chopped
2–3 celery stalks, chopped
½ pound of fresh green peas from the pod

Put all ingredients except vegetables in a blender and blend until very smooth. Add the steamed or steam-fried vegetables and serve warm. This soup is even better the next day. Store in the refrigerator overnight so the flavors blend.

RECIPES FOR USE DURING A LIQUID FEAST OR CLEANSE

(Any of the cleanse recipes from the other pH Miracle books could also be used.)

(continued)

SALADS

Alkalarian Coleslaw

Contributed by Sheila Mack

SERVES 4–6

½ head green cabbage, shredded
2 medium carrots, shredded
½ small red onion, sliced thinly into strips
½ cup chopped Italian parsley

Dressing

1 cup coconut milk (make it fresh by blending the coconut water
    and meat of a Thai coconut in a blender)
1 tsp. arrowroot powder to thicken (if needed)
½ tsp. sea salt or to taste
¼ tsp. celery seed
Dash of cayenne pepper
2 Tbs. fresh lime juice

Place first four ingredients into a bowl and toss. Blend coconut milk and arrowroot. Add seasonings and lime juice. Blend. Pour over cabbage mixture. Toss and enjoy!

Optional: Add a little stevia if you need it a bit sweeter. Also, chilling this recipe and letting it sit makes the flavors blend even better.

Cabbage Delight

Contributed by Linda Broadhead
Third place, pH Miracle 2004 Recipe Contest
Transitional Category

SERVES 6

1 red cabbage, chopped
2 scallions, white only
½ cup pure water
1 Tbs. grapeseed oil
2 Tbs. toasted sesame oil
2 Tbs. olive oil
Pinch stevia
Juice of ½ lemon
¼ tsp. RealSalt
¼ cup cilantro, chopped
½ cup pine nuts
2 scallions, greens
½ cup cooked quinoa

Steam-fry half of the chopped cabbage and the whites of scallions in water and grapeseed oil, until wilted. Mix other ingredients including remaining cabbage. Stir into wilted cabbage. Serve warm or cold.

Crispy Oriental Salad

Contributed by Cristianne Casper
Third place, pH Miracle 2004 Recipe Contest
Transitional Category

SERVES 4–8

Salad

1–2 heads lettuce, shredded
4 green onions, diced
1 cup almonds, soaked and diced
¼ cup sesame seeds

Dressing

1–2 drops liquid stevia or 1 packet stevia
1 tsp. RealSalt
½ tsp. pepper
4 Tbs. lemon juice
¼ cup sesame oil
¼ cup grapeseed oil or oil of choice

Mix salad ingredients together.
Mix dressing ingredients with whisk. Pour over salad just before serving.

Dream Castle Salad

Contributed by Lisa El-Kerdi
Best in Show, pH Miracle 2004 Recipe Contest

SERVES 6–12

Use 1 artichoke bottom per person for first course or 2 for entrée. If using canned, be sure to buy bottoms rather than quartered hearts.
With scissors, cut dried tomato halves into strips. Place in glass jar with good-quality olive oil. This should be done at least a week in advance and stored in a cool, dark cupboard.

Flags (optional)

4-inch piece of foil wrapping paper (optional)
Craft glue
Colored toothpicks (optional)

To make flags, cut small triangles and squares out of foil wrapping paper (2 flags per person). Vary colors if possible. Apply thin strip of craft glue to colored toothpick (width of flag) and wrap end of paper around pick.

6–12 artichoke bottoms, fresh (simmer until just tender) or canned
¼ cup lemon juice
1 bay leaf, celery stalk, rind of ½ lemon
12 squash blossoms or 2 red and 2 yellow bell peppers, julienne
1–2 fat carrots, shaved thinly into lengths and cut into fish shapes
1–1½ lbs. baby salad greens
1–2 small heads radicchio, shredded
1 lb. sunflower sprouts
Paté Bernaise (page 276)
1 cup dried tomatoes, julienned and soaked in olive oil (see above)
2–3 avocados, sliced
Lemon and Tomato Dressing (recipe follows)

Rinse and dry canned artichoke bottoms and coat with lemon juice to freshen. If using fresh artichokes, cut leaves off halfway down. Place in pot of salted water with 1 bay leaf, 1 celery stalk, and rind of half a lemon. Bring to a boil, simmer, covered until bottoms are just tender (½ to 1 hour). Remove from pot, cool, and gently remove leaves and hairy choke. Coat with lemon juice. May be cooked day before, waiting until serving day to remove leaves. If using bell peppers, slice in half horizontally, and remove seeds before slicing into thin vertical strips. Peppers may also be roasted and skins removed before slicing. Prepare carrots. Make lengthwise shavings with vegetable peeler, stack, and cut into small fish shapes. Soak in ice water in fridge until assembly.

First Course Assembly for Salad

Place small circular bed of greens in center of salad plate for dream castle island and a small circle to one side of plate for a tea house island. Surround castle island (main island) with a "wall" of shredded radicchio (optional). First course will have one castle with one teahouse. Place sunflower sprouts around large island to symbolize water. Place artichoke bottom in center of large island. Place a mound (approx. ¼ cup) of Paté Bernaise on artichoke and a small mound to create castle turret. Place second blossom on small teahouse mound. Carefully open petals of squash blossom and arrange on top of mound, having them meet at the top and fan out around the bottom to create turret. Or, if using peppers, place alternating strips of red and yellow on both mounds, having them meet at the top and fan out at the bottom to form the turret. Sprinkle oil-soaked tomato "fish" and carrot "goldfish" on sunflower sprout moat. Place "bridge" of avocado slices between castle island and teahouse island. Drizzle dressing over salad. Place flag (optional, see note) in top of each turret. Dream away!

Mung Bean Sprout and Avocado Salad

Contributed by Marlene Grauwels
First place, pH Miracle 2004 Recipe Contest
Alkalizing Category

SERVES 4–6

1 cup sprouted mung beans
1–2 avocados, diced
1–2 tomatoes, diced
1 lime, juiced
Fresh basil to taste
¼ cup olive oil, or Arrowhead Mills Ideal Balance oil
Herbamare to taste

Mix all ingredients.

Variation:
  • Add any of the following chopped: asparagus, jicama, or your
    favorite.

Popeye Salmon Salad

Contributed by Maraline Krey
First place, pH Miracle 2004 Recipe Contest
Alkalizing Category

SERVES 4

1½ lbs. salmon fillet (cold water preferred) (salmon is optional)
1 lemon
1 lime
4 oz. distilled water

Popeye Salad

1 lb. spinach leaves
½ cup basil leaves
1 cup hearts of palm, diced
1 cup carrots, diced (optional)
1 cup celery, diced (optional)
1 cup tomato, diced (optional)
1 cup asparagus, diced (optional)

Salad Dressing

2 limes
2 oz. avocado oil or extra-virgin olive oil
Ground pepper
RealSalt
1 oz. ground flaxseed
1 oz. poppy seed
Handful of pine nuts (optional)

Preheat the oven to 400 degrees Fahrenheit. Place salmon fillet in a glass baking dish. In a bowl, squeeze lemon and lime juice, add water, and stir. Pour mixture over salmon, marinade for 1 hour, flip salmon and marinade another hour. (If you are in a time crunch, place in a Ziploc bag and let soak in refrigerator for half an hour.) Bake salmon in the citrus/water mixture for 30 minutes at 400 degrees F. Last 5 minutes put under broiler to brown top, creating a steaming effect (for crispy edges). For the salad dressing: Roll limes on counter to soften before squeezing into a mixing bowl, add the oil, stir in pepper and RealSalt, then flax and poppy seeds and optional pine nuts. For the salad: Cut spinach and basil with kitchen scissors (the size of baby spinach leaves) into a large salad bowl. Add all diced ingredients, then salad dressing. Set aside. To serve pour the dressing over the salad, toss, and place a generous serving on each plate, covering the plate. Break up salmon and place pieces over the salad—beautiful!

Variation:
- This can also be served with Rustic Guacamole, found in Shelley's book *Back to the House of Health 2.*

Rainbow Salad

SERVES 8–12

I love the colors of the vegetables! Presentation of a beautifully arranged alkalizing meal can be an art. Besides, eating a rainbow of colored foods supports the balance of the energy of the body. This salad is my basic salad recipe that I make every week. The grating of the vegetables exposes their natural sweetness.

1–2 heads green-leaf lettuce, washed, dried, ripped into bite-sized pieces
1–2 heads red-leaf lettuce, washed, rinsed, dried, ripped into bite-sized pieces
1 pkg. prewashed baby leaf organic spinach
1 head green cabbage, shredded
½–1 head red cabbage, shredded
3–4 beets, grated
4–5 carrots, grated
2–3 summer squash, or zucchini, grated, or ½ butternut squash, grated
⅓–½ jicama, grated
1 each red, yellow, orange bell peppers, sliced
1–2 cucumbers, sliced
1–2 pkgs. (8 oz) sunflower seeds sprouts, or sprout mix of choice
1 lb. fresh green peas from the pod
1–2 Tbs. salad dressing of your choice, per serving

Fill a large salad bowl with the lettuces, spinach, and cabbages. Packaged lettuce mixes are fine if very fresh and organic. Arrange grated vegetables on top of the greens, starting with the deeper colored vegetables on outside, in a half circle. Continue rainbow color sequencing with vegetables within the crescent being formed. Place bell pepper and cucumber slices at top of plate. Sprinkle with sprouts and peas. Top with dressing and pass extra dressing at table. Or just sprinkle spices to taste, Bragg Liquid Aminos, a healthy oil, and fresh lemon juice.

Soba Cabbage Salad

Contributed by Ashley Lisonbee

SERVES 8–10

1 head cabbage, chopped
4 green onions, chopped
2 Tbs. sesame seeds, toasted
¾ cup chopped almonds, toasted
1 Tbs. grapeseed oil
½ pkg. soba noodles, buckwheat (Eden)

Dressing

½ cup grapeseed oil
1 medium grapefruit or lime juice
3 Tbs. vegetable dehydrated mix
½ tsp. salt
Dash of stevia to taste

Chop cabbage into bite-sized pieces and mix with green onions. Place sesame seeds and chopped almonds in a pan with grapeseed oil and gently toast on medium heat. Bring soba noodles and water to a boil for 4 to 5 minutes. Remove from heat and cut into bite-sized noodle pieces with kitchen scissors. Mix together the cabbage, nuts, and noodles into one bowl. In a separate bowl mix the dressing ingredients and add to the salad, toss well. Enjoy!

Variation:
- Add flavored baked tofu if desired.

Summer Pad Thai Salad

Contributed by Lisa El-Kerdi
Best in Show, pH Miracle 2004 Recipe Contest

SERVES 6–8

1 spaghetti squash, baked
3 green onions including tops, thinly sliced
1 carrot, shredded
1 jalapeño pepper, minced
1 red bell pepper, thinly sliced and cut into fourths lengthwise
3 cups broccoli crowns, thinly sliced
2 stalks celery, minced or thinly sliced
2–3 cups snow peas, trimmed and sliced into ½-inch pieces
4 Tbs. cilantro, leaves only, chopped
4 Tbs. mint leaves, chopped (optional)
½ cup sliced almonds, soaked and dehydrated if possible
1 English cucumber, peeled, seeded, and cubed
Black sesame seeds plus extra for garnish
Sunflower sprouts (for top)

Pad Thai Dressing

2-inch piece of gingerroot, peeled and sliced
2 large garlic cloves
1 tsp. crushed red pepper flakes (adjust to taste)
½ cup Bragg Liquid Aminos

½ **cup lime juice**
⅔ **cup raw tahini**
½ **cup crunchy almond butter**
½ **cup cold-pressed, unrefined sesame oil**
2 **Tbs. toasted sesame oil**

Bake squash the night before. Bake until slightly softened but still firm, approximately 30 to 45 minutes. Remove seeds and pull strands into "spaghetti" strands with a fork. Refrigerate. The day of serving, prepare vegetables. When ready to serve, toss squash, remaining ingredients, and enough dressing to coat. Reserve sprouts and some black sesame seeds for top garnish. For the dressing: Blend first three ingredients in food processor or Vita-Mix. Add Bragg Liquid Aminos and lime juice. Blend until smooth. Blend in tahini and almond butter. Slowly add oils with motor running. Refrigerate until ready to use.

Sunshine Salad and Dressing

Contributed by Frances Parkton
Second place, pH Miracle 2003 Recipe Contest

SERVES 6–8

2 **cups quinoa, cooked**
1 **cup zucchini, minced**
2 **cups broccoli, minced**
1 **cup onion, minced**
1 **red or orange bell pepper, minced**
1 **cup pine nuts**
2 **Tbs. toasted sesame oil**
Salt to taste
Tomatoes, chopped to taste
Parsley, minced to taste

Sunshine Dressing

2 cups cucumber
2 sun-dried tomatoes
1 cup onions, minced
4 jalepeño peppers, minced
1 cup olive oil
½ cup avocado oil
¼ cup veganaise (non-vinegar)
2 limes, juiced
2 tsps. Mexican seasoning
2 tsps. Herbamare (A. Vogel)
½ tsp. cayenne pepper
2 tsps. garlic, minced

Combine all ingredients except the dressing in a bowl.
For the dressing: In a blender, on low speed to start, blend all the dressing ingredients except seasonings. Increase speed to make smooth. Add and adjust seasonings to taste. Toss with salad.

Tera's Hearty Party

Contributed by Tera Prestwich

SERVES 4–6

1 head of broccoli
1 head of cauliflower
2 celery stalks, sliced
3 green onions
1 red bell pepper
1 green bell pepper
1 orange bell pepper
1 (12 oz.) bag of edamame (soy beans)
½ cup Essential Balance Oil (or oil of choice)

½ garlic clove, minced
¼ cup of Bragg Liquid Aminos or 1–2 tsp. RealSalt
1 Tbs. Garlic Herb Bread Seasoning (Spice Hunter)
Zip (Spice Hunter) for garnish

Chop up broccoli, cauliflower, celery, green onions, and bell peppers. Mix together. Cook edamame as directed and add to mix. Add in the Essential Oil, minced garlic, Bragg Liquid Aminos, and Garlic Herb Bread Seasoning. Toss together and garnish with Zip.

Tofu Potato Salad/Stuffed in Tomato Blossom

Contributed by Victoria's Gourmet—Victoria Frerichs
Professional Award, pH Miracle 2004 Recipe Contest

1 large tomato for each serving
Packaged extra-firm tofu, cubed (¼ cup per tomato)

Wash tomatoes. Cut three times down from top only ¾ into tomato (leaving the bottom of the tomato whole) forming the "blossom."

Dressing

1 lemon, juiced
1 cup oil
1 packet stevia
1 tsp. dry mustard
Celery, chopped to taste
Green onion, chopped to taste
Dill, to taste
Zip to taste

Press tofu in glass pan as follows: Drain tofu. Layer tofu slice, four layers of paper towels, tofu slice, paper towels, paper plate, cans or books to add weight. Leave overnight in fridge. Cut in cubes as you would for potato salad. For dressing, whisk until thickened, adjust seasonings. Add celery, onion, and dill. Toss with tofu. Chill 3 hours. Sprinkle with Zip (Spice Hunter) to add taste and color. Fill tomato with tofu and dressing mixture. Serve.

Zucchini Salad

Contributed by Linnette Webster
First place, pH Miracle 2004 Recipe Contest
Transitional Category

SERVES 4–6

**4 zucchinis, large
1 cup pumpkin, sesame, and sunflower seed combination
1 cup millet or spelt flour
RealSalt to taste
1 Tbs. olive oil**

Slice zucchinis into half-inch slices. In a coffee grinder, grind the seed combination, ¼ cup at a time. Combine ground seeds, flour, and salt in a mixing bowl. Coat zucchini slices with mixture. In a skillet, heat olive oil, then brown zucchini on each side. Add a small amount of water, cover, and steam-fry 4 minutes. Layer zucchini slices in a bowl with your favorite dressing. Cover and refrigerate 24 hours before serving.

DRESSINGS, DIPS, AND SAUCES

Casper's Ranch Dressing

Contributed by Cristianne Casper
Third place, pH Miracle 2004 Recipe Contest
Transitional Category

MAKES 2 QUARTS

1 qt. milk (almond, soy, or sesame)
1 qt. Mock Mayo (found in Shelley's book *Back to the House of Health*)
¾ tsp. pepper
2½ tsps. RealSalt
2 tsps. onion salt
½ tsp. garlic powder
2 tsps. parsley, chopped

Mix all ingredients together in blender. Refrigerate for half hour before using. For thicker dressing use less milk.

Chipotle Chili Pepper Sauce

Contributed by Linnette Webster
First place, pH Miracle 2004 Recipe Contest
Transitional Category

3 tomatoes
½ tsp. Chipotle Chili Pepper (Spice Hunter), crushed
¹/₁₆ tsp. stevia
1 garlic clove, minced
2 tsps. RealSalt
Water to desired consistency

Blend ingredients, adding enough water to make medium thick sauce.

Variations:
- Serve as soup. Add sauce to vegetables with just enough water to desired consistency. Warm to serve.
- Serve in a pre-baked pumpkin (golden nugget squash), cut top, remove seeds and oil. Bake at 350 degrees F for 30 minutes.
- Serve as vegetable dish with sauce and tofu.

Creamy Cilantro Lime Dressing

Contributed by Cristianne Casper
Third place, pH Miracle 2004 Recipe Contest
Transitional Category

MAKES 2 CUPS

1 cup mock mayo
¾ cup fresh almond milk
½ jalepeño pepper, seeded and chopped
1 cup cilantro leaves, loosely packed
3 Tbs. lime juice
1 garlic clove, peeled
½ tsp. RealSalt
½-inch piece fresh ginger, peeled, chopped

Mix all ingredients in blender. Store in refrigerator.

Esther's All-Purpose Dressing

Contributed by Esther Andreas
Third place, pH Miracle 2004 Recipe Contest
Alkalizing Category

MAKES 1 QUART

1 bunch green onions or ¼ cup white onions
1 cup water and 1 tsp. RealSalt (or ½ cup water and ½ cup Nama
  Shoyu or Bragg Liquid Aminos)
Pinch of cayenne pepper to taste
½ cup lemon juice
¼–½ packet stevia to taste
3 Tbs. raw tahini or raw hemp butter
1 tsp. gingerroot
2 cups olive oil

Blend all the ingredients in a blender on high until creamy. Great as sauce on quinoa, rice, buckwheat, or Esther's Hearty Sprouted Lentil Burgers (page 296).

Esther's Creamy Mayo

Contributed by Esther Andreas
Third place, pH Miracle 2004 Recipe Contest
Alkalizing Category

MAKES 1¼ CUPS

Save milk of coconut used in recipe to drink!

2 fresh young coconuts (meat only)
2 Tbs. lemon juice
½ tsp. RealSalt
¼ tsp. mild mustard powder

½ tsp. garlic powder
¾ cup olive oil

Blend all ingredients except olive oil. Slowly drizzle oil into mixture while blending. Store in refrigerator, with airtight lid.

Garlic French Dressing

Contributed by Myra Marvez Corbett
Second place, pH Miracle 2004 Recipe Contest
Transitional Category

MAKES 2–3 CUPS

½ cup dried tomato
1 lemon, juiced
3 garlic cloves
1 tsp. RealSalt
1 tsp. paprika
½ tsp. cayenne
1–2 packets stevia
2 cups pure water

Blend all ingredients in blender until smooth and creamy.
Note: Up to 20 oz. of water may be added.

Herbed Alkalarian Butter

SERVES 6–8

You can always put different oils (Udo's, flax, olive, and Essential Balance) on your steamed veggies and warmed grains, or in your wraps, but now through the inspiration of Dr. Johanna Budwig, who was a great advocate of the healing properties of flaxseed oil, I have discovered a combination of healthy oils and herbed seasonings that is the alkaline answer to butter. It makes a solid spread but melts beautifully once it hits something warm. Coconut oil keeps it solid in the fridge, and flax oil gives it a rich golden appearance. Experiment with different herbs, spices, and flavorings.

Do not cook or fry with this herbed alkalarian butter as the heat will cause trans-fatty acids to form. Keep the mixture raw and use only after you have cooked or warmed your food. Great on the Zippy Breakfast (found in The pH Miracle*)!*

1 cup coconut oil (Wilderness Family Naturals) (I use Organic Extra Virgin cold-pressed)
1 yellow onion
8 large garlic cloves
½–1 tsp. RealSalt
2 tsps. Italian seasoning (Spice Hunter) or your choice
1 tsp. fresh rosemary, minced
2 tsps. sun-dried tomatoes, minced (optional)
½ cup Barlean's Flax Oil (in the refrigerated section of your natural food store)

In a nonstick pan, heat 3 Tbs. of the coconut oil. Sauté diced onion and garlic until onion is clear, stirring constantly. If desired, slightly brown the onions and garlic for a more roasted flavor. Add remaining coconut oil, letting it melt until clear. Stir to mix. Take off burner, do not cook. Strain the mixture through a strainer to take out the pieces of onion and garlic or if desired leave them in. Add salt, spices, and seasonings of choice and the Barlean's Flax Oil. Stir mix well, pour into small tubs, and place into the refrigerator to set up.

Variations:
- Add lemon juice to tang it up.
- Use Frontier Herb Flavorings (bottled without alcohol) to enhance the taste. Example: Mint or put fresh mint minced in the butter.
- Add diced pecans or almonds to make a more nutty butter.

Hot, Sweet Poppy Seed Dressing

SERVES 4

1 cup of Essential Balance Dressing (Arrowhead Mills or Omega Nutrition)
1–2 tsps. of Olivado Gold avocado oil (infused with chili and bell pepper—you can order this beautiful avocado oil from Bio-Grow, www.YourNatureStore.com)
2 large limes, juiced
1 lemon, juiced
1 pkg. stevia (I use Sweetleaf with fiber)
1 oz. ground yellow flaxseed (I use a small coffee grinder to grind this small amount)
¼ cup raw pine nuts or raw macadamia nuts
Ground pepper or Zip (Spice Hunter) to taste
½–1 tsp. RealSalt to taste
1 oz. poppy seeds

Add the first seven ingredients in a Cuisinart food processor. Blend until ground flaxseed is well mixed and begins to thicken. With processor running, add pepper (or Zip) and RealSalt (stopping to adjust the seasoning). Add the poppy seeds and blend for a couple of seconds to mix.

This dressing is even better and thicker if allowed to chill in refrigerator.

K&L Poppy Seed Dressing

Contributed by Linnette Webster
First place, pH Miracle 2004 Recipe Contest
Transitional Category

MAKES ¾ CUP

½ cup soymilk, unsweetened (Westsoy)
¼ tsp. dry mustard
2 Tbs. lemon juice
Salt to taste
¼ tsp. paprika
6 Tbs. olive oil, mild flavor
1 Tbs. poppy seeds

In blender, combine all ingredients (except poppy seeds) until smooth. Fold in poppy seeds.

K&L Ranch Dressing

Contributed by Linnette Webster
First place, pH Miracle 2004 Recipe Contest
Transitional Category

MAKES ¾ CUP

½ cup soymilk, unsweetened (Westsoy)
6 Tbs. olive oil, mild flavor
2 Tbs. lemon juice
3 Tbs. green onion, chopped
1 Tbs. parsley, chopped
¼ tsp. dry mustard
1 tsp. onion powder
¼ tsp. paprika
¼ tsp. RealSalt
⅛ tsp. red pepper
$1/_{16}$ tsp. white stevia

In blender, combine all ingredients until smooth.

K&L Thousand Island Dressing

Contributed by Linnette Webster
First place, pH Miracle 2004 Recipe Contest
Transitional Category

MAKES ¾ CUP

½ cup soymilk, unsweetened (Westsoy)
¼ tsp. dry mustard
1 Tbs. lemon juice
½ tsp. salt
1¼ tsps. paprika
6 Tbs. olive oil, mild flavor
$^1/_{16}$ tsp. stevia or to taste
2 sun-dried tomatoes, packed in olive oil
1 Tbs. each: onion, chopped; green pepper, chopped; celery, chopped

In blender, combine all ingredients until smooth.

Lemon and Tomato Dressing

Contributed by Lisa El-Kerdi
Best in Show, pH Miracle 2004 Recipe Contest

MAKES 1 CUP

⅓ cup lemon juice
¾ cup olive oil from oil-soaked tomatoes
½ tsp. RealSalt
Black pepper, freshly ground

Whisk or blend all ingredients together.

Lemon Basil Dressing

Contributed by Victoria's Gourmet—Victoria Frerichs
Professional Award, pH Miracle 2004 Recipe Contest

MAKES ABOUT 1½ CUPS

**1 lemon, grated finely, and juice
3 Tbs. fresh basil, finely minced
Dash stevia
Salt to taste
1 block of tofu
1 cup olive oil**

Mix first four ingredients until blended. Puree with tofu. Whisk in oil.

Lisa's Elegant Sauces

Contributed by Lisa El-Kerdi
Best in Show, pH Miracle 2004 Recipe Contest

Basic Hollandaise Sauce

**1 large garlic clove
1½ tsps. RealSalt
½ cup lemon juice
½ tsp. paprika
½ tsp. dry mustard
⅛ tsp. cayenne
1 green onion, bulb and top
1½–2 celery stalks
½ cup sunflower seeds, soaked for 6–8 hours
1½ cups olive oil**

Combine garlic and salt in food processor. Add lemon juice and spices. Blend. Add all remaining ingredients except olive oil and blend. "Slowly" drizzle in olive oil with food processor running. Blend until smooth.

Variation:

Lemon Version
- Use ¾–1 cup lemon juice instead of ½ cup. All sauces can be made in regular or lemony versions. For extra kick add 1 tsp. lemon rind.

Paté Bernaise

For paté or spread, make any of these recipes using this base and add appropriate seasonings. Delicious as a vegetable dip or spread for wraps, tortillas, or nori rolls.

2 cups sunflower seeds, soaked 6–8 hours
1½ cups almonds, soaked 6–8 hours
½ cup walnuts, soaked 6–8 hours
3 garlic cloves
2 cups celery
1 tsp. RealSalt
½ cup lemon juice
1½ cups olive oil
Herbs and seasonings (see recipes)

Variations:

Aioli
Increase garlic clove to 3 or more to taste.
For roasted garlic aioli, roast 1 head of garlic and substitute 6 to 8 cloves for fresh garlic.
For red pepper aioli, add ½ cup roasted red pepper to either of the above.
Add ½ cup sun-dried tomato and ½ cup fresh or 1 tsp. dried basil.

Bernaise

Add ½–1 tsp. crushed dried tarragon to Basic Hollandaise sauce.

Curry Sauce

Omit mustard in Basic Hollandaise sauce and add ½–1 tsp. curry powder.

French Herb Sauce

Omit mustard in Basic Hollandaise Sauce and add ½ cup fresh parsley, ½ cup fresh chives, and 1 to 2 tsps. crushed dried Herbes de Provence.

Caesar Dressing

Make Lemon Version Hollandaise using 2 cups olive oil, 2 to 3 garlic cloves, and ¾ cup lemon juice. Add 1 tsp. crushed dried oregano and freshly ground pepper. Blend, leaving dressing a little coarse rather than a smooth puree.

Southwest Caesar Dressing

Using Caesar Dressing recipe, substitute lime juice for lemon juice. Add 1 tsp. red chili powder, ⅓ tsp. cumin (and original 1 tsp. oregano).

Green Goddess Dressing

Make Caesar Dressing (without oregano) using Lemon Version Bernaise as a base.

Add 1 cup parsley, 1 more green onion, and 1 tsp. Bragg Liquid Aminos. Blend until smooth.

Nut Variations: Alter flavor of any of the above by substituting various nuts for the sunflower seeds. Try 2 Tbs. sunflower seeds, 2 Tbs. soaked almonds, and 2 Tbs. soaked walnuts.

MamaGrand's French Dressing

SERVES 4–6

1½ cups oil of choice (I use Barlean's Flax, Udo's, olive,
    or grapeseed)
2 lemons, juiced
1 lime, juiced

Shake in the following spices to taste or use the following measurements:

1 tsp. Grill and Broil (Spice Hunter)
½ tsp. Zip (Spice Hunter)
¼ tsp. dry mustard
½–1 tsp. garlic powder or garlic salt (Spice Hunter)
Pinch of Deliciously Dill (Spice Hunter)
RealSalt to taste
½ red bell pepper
1 tomato
½ cucumber (I use English)
1 Tbs. flaxseeds to thicken

In blender or food processor, place oil and lemon/lime juice mix. With machine running add spices. Add remaining vegetables in the order given and blend to desired consistency. Add flaxseed, blend. Flaxseeds will thicken dressing even more if chilled overnight.

Pepita Seed Dressing

Contributed by Victoria's Gourmet—Victoria Frerichs
Professional Award, pH Miracle 2004 Recipe Contest

MAKES 1½ CUPS

1 cup green raw pepita seeds
1 cup Basic Lemon Vinaigrette (recipe follows)

Toast seeds lightly in oven on dry pan. Blend with Basic Lemon Vinaigrette. Reserve 1 Tbs. whole pepita seed to garnish each salad.

Basic Lemon Vinaigrette

3 parts olive oil
1 part lemon juice
Salt and Zip to taste

Mix oil and lemon juice thoroughly. Add salt and Zip to taste.

Sesame Soy (Bragg) Dressing

Contributed by Victoria's Gourmet—Victoria Frerichs
Professional Award, pH Miracle 2004 Recipe Contest

Bragg Liquid Aminos
Stevia
Garlic powder
Zip

Blend first three ingredients to taste. Add Zip to taste.

Simply Alkalarian Salad Dressings/Sauces/Dips

Quick and Easy Make to Taste

Contributed by Maraline Krey
First place, pH Miracle 2004 Recipe Contest
Alkalizing Category

This array of tasty shortcuts and tasty tidbits are for Alkalarians who have little time but very big appetites for the Alkalarian lifestyle. Maraline says: "Let's not 'substitute,' but let us 'replace' with better tasting, better for you, and, most important, better results!"

Simply Salad Dressings

Basic

Squeeze lime or lemon into a dish. Add equal parts avocado oil, virgin coconut oil, or olive oil. Sprinkle with spices of choice. Whisk and toss your salad.

Basic Plus:　Add one or more of the following

Avocado, puree
½ sesame oil and ½ other oil of choice
Ginger, puree
Tahini, puree
Garlic and onion, puree
Tofutti cream cheese, puree
Almond butter and cayenne pepper, puree

Simple Salads

Each week add a new and interesting ingredient to your selection. Prepare at least two different dressings for variety.

Veggies
Purchase weekly (twice a week if time allows), wash in baking soda water, cut roughly into thirds, and store in large bowl covered with water.

Lettuce and Herbs
Scissor or tear, but don't "wash" until ready to use. Store open in drawer or in plastic bags with holes.

Simple Spreads for Wraps

Use Boston-type lettuce for wrap, Nori squares, or healthy tortillas. Toss in diced veggies and/or layer with rice.

Ginger/Pepper Spread

1 red bell pepper
1 Tbs. ginger
1 Tbs. coconut oil
RealSalt to taste

Puree in blender.

Tahini Bean Hummus Spread

1 cup white kidney beans or garbanzo beans
2 Tbs. tahini
2 oz. tofu
¼ lime or lemon, juiced

Puree in blender

Variations:
- Add any of the following for variety: bell pepper, eggplant, garlic, cinnamon, herbs of choice (i.e., basil, cilantro, parsley).
- Layer grated veggies with avocado.

Creamy Soft Spread

4 oz. Tofuttti cream cheese
4 oz. soft tofu
1 Tbs. tahini

Blend, refrigerate after use.

Simple Sauces or Dips

Serve with flax chips, veggies, rice, fish, or quinoa pasta.

Artichoke Pesto Sauces or Dip

10–12 artichoke hearts
½ lemon, juiced
¼ cup avocado or olive oil

Blend.

Grapefruit/Avocado Salsa

1 grapefruit, sectioned
1 avocado, diced
Cilantro to taste
Onion, diced, to taste
Garlic, diced, to taste
RealSalt to taste

Mix.

Variation:
• Tomatoes can be substituted for grapefruit.

Alkalarian Teriyaki Sauce

¼ cup Bragg Liquid Aminos, or to taste
1 tsp. ginger, pureed, or to taste
1 pkg. stevia, to taste (such as Sweet Leaf brand with fiber)
⅛ pure water, or to taste
1 Tbs. sesame oil
1 tsp. arrowroot

Warm in saucepan coated with sesame oil. Sauce can be thickened with arrowroot.

Almond Thai Sauce

⅓ cup almond butter
1 Tbs. coconut oil
⅓ cup coconut milk
Cayenne to taste
Sesame oil

Warm in saucepan coated with sesame oil. Sauce can be thickened with more almond butter.

Walla Rice Bowls

Assorted vegetables
2 cups Alkalarian Sauce base (any suggested sauce base)
Add veggies to sauce base. Cook over low heat (Crock-Pot on low is best). Ready when veggies are still chunky but sauce is thickened. Great over rice!

Spicy Southwestern Chipotle Sauce

Contributed by Sheila Mack

MAKES 1½ CUPS

I use this spicy sauce in wraps, to top veggies and fish. I also use it as a dip or salad dressing.

½ cup raw pine nuts (soak a minimum 2 hours and discard water)
1 medium clove garlic
1 Tbs. fresh lime juice
2–3 sun-dried tomatoes (softened in warm water)
1 small tomato, quartered
1 medium red pepper, roasted
½–1 tsp. crushed Chipotle Chile Pepper (Spice Hunter)
¼ tsp. Mesquite Seasoning (Spice Hunter)
½–¾ tsp. RealSalt
⅛ cup onion

Put all ingredients into a blender or processor. Begin blending ingredients while slowly adding ¼ cup olive oil to emulsify. Sauce will be thick and creamy. Garnish with chopped cilantro.
Note: For added nutrition, add 1–2 scoops of Super Soy Sprout Powder.

Sun-Dried Tomato Spread

Contributed by Michael Steadman
Second place, pH Miracle 2004 Recipe Contest
Transitional Category

MAKES 2 CUPS

2 cups sun-dried tomatoes
1 cup olive oil

12 garlic cloves
1 Tbs. dried basil
¼ tsp. cayenne
1 tsp. Celtic Salt or ¾ tsp. RealSalt
1 packet stevia or equivalent

Pour boiling water over tomatoes to rehydrate. Let sit for 5 minutes. Squeeze out excess water. Chop into small strips. In food processor, pulse-chop all ingredients, blending until smooth. Store in refrigerator.

Super Soy Seaweed Dressing

SERVES 4

This is a versatile dressing that can be made thick for a dip, or thinned out for a dressing. Hiziki is a dried seaweed you can usually find in the macrobiotic section of your natural food store. For the nuts in the recipe, I use fresh organic macadamias from Jaffe's Bros. (see Resources) and crack them fresh. Jaffe's Bros. also sell a terrific nutcracker that breaks the hard shells with ease.

1 cup macadamia nuts, freshly cracked
1 large lime, juiced
2 scoops Super Soy Powder
1 clove garlic
2 Tbs. dry Hiziki seaweed
½ cup coconut water (taken from a Thai coconut)
½ cup water, to thin to desired consistency
Pinch of Zip (Spice Hunter)

Blend all ingredients in Vita-Mix blender until smooth and creamy. Thin with more coconut water or water if desired. I use this recipe as a dip for the Tofu Italian Mock Meatballs (found in Shelley's book *Back to the House of Health*).

Tomato Basil Sauce

Contributed by Lorie Lisonbee

Serves 4–6

4 Tbs. olive oil
4 garlic cloves, minced
1 onion, chopped
4 cups tomatoes, chopped
2 bunches fresh basil, without stems
⅛ tsp. crushed red pepper
Salt and pepper to taste
½ cup coconut or almond milk (optional)

In a skillet, heat oil and sauté garlic and onion until tender. Add the tomatoes, basil, and spices. Simmer for 15 to 20 minutes. In food processor, blend sauce until desired consistency. Add coconut milk or almond milk to make a creamier sauce. Enjoy over steamed vegetables or baked spaghetti squash.

ENTRÉES/SIDE DISHES

Artichoke Pesto Pasta

Contributed by Maraline Krey
First place, pH Miracle 2004 Recipe Contest
Alkalizing Category

SERVES 4

Artichoke Pesto

½ lemon, juiced
¼ cup avocado oil or coconut oil
10–12 artichoke hearts (frozen, fresh, or packed in water)

Vegetables

1 cucumber, seeded and sliced lengthwise
2 cups baby spinach leaves
½ lime, juiced
1½ Tbs. avocado oil or coconut oil (optional olive oil)

Pasta

3 qts. water
2 Tbs. grapeseed oil or coconut oil
1 (8 oz.) package quinoa linguini, cooked and drained
2 Tbs. avocado oil
¼ cup vegetable broth
1 tsp. RealSalt
1 tsp. organic pepper
¼ cup basil, scissor cut

Pesto Prep. In food processor, puree lemon and oil. Pulse-chop artichokes into mixture until just blended, leaving pesto "chunky."

Vegetable Prep. Chop cucumber. Toss with spinach. Combine lime juice and oil, add to cucumbers and spinach to marinate.

Pasta Prep. Bring 3 quarts of water to a boil and add 2 Tbs. oil. Add pasta, stirring constantly. Cook 4 to 6 minutes (don't overcook).

   Drain, place back into pot. Toss with avocado oil, broth, salt, pepper, and basil.

Presentation: Layer on plate:

Tossed spinach and cucumber with dressing, pasta with basil, artichoke pesto over top.

Artichokes Stuffed with Pesto/Variations

Contributed by Mary Jo and George Walter
Honorable Mention, pH Miracle 2004 Recipe Contest

PESTO MAKES 1 CUP

1 artichoke per person
1 garlic clove, sliced into slivers
1 lemon, sliced

Pesto

2 Tbs. pine nuts
3 garlic cloves
2 cups basil, loosely packed
4 green onions, cut in 1-inch pieces
¼ tsp. RealSalt
¼ tsp. white pepper
2 Tbs. extra-virgin olive oil
¼ cup distilled water

Preheat the oven to 350 degrees F. Prepare artichokes by soaking and rinsing in water. With scissors, trim thorny edges of leaves. Slice ¼ to ½ inch off top center point and cut stem to ½ inch. Prepare ovenproof dish. Slip a sliver of garlic into leaves in five places around artichoke. Place ¼ cup water and a lemon slice per artichoke in baking dish. For the pesto: In food processor, pulse-chop pine nuts and garlic. Add basil, onion, salt, and pepper. Pulse until finely chopped. Drizzle in olive oil and water, process until well mixed, scraping down sides of container often. Taste, adjust seasoning, blend to mix. Adjust consistency by adding more pine nuts. Spoon 2 Tbs. pesto sauce into top center and rub lightly around side leaves of artichoke. Bake for 35 to 45 minutes. Artichoke is done when leaves pull away easily. Carefully remove and trim artichoke stem so it will stand up on plate. Spoon the sauce from bottom of dish over top of artichoke.

Variation:

- Grilling artichokes in a foil pouch is an alternate cooking method.
- Pesto sauce can be used warm, over spelt pasta (dressed with olive oil). Also add chopped tomatoes, green onion, and celery. Mix with pasta and chill in refrigerator for great cool pasta dish.
- Bake salmon and place on bed of spinach. Top with warmed pesto.
- Make cheese substitute: drain white kidney beans, mash into puree. Add pesto until desired consistency. Adjust seasoning to taste. Serve as topping on vegetable combinations such as roasted zucchini and green and red bell peppers. Or top roasted asparagus, or crisp-fried eggplant and tomatoes.

Asian Bean Sprouts

Contributed by Raye Haskell

SERVES 2

½ cup green onion, chopped
1 garlic clove
¼ cup pure water
1 cup mung bean sprouts
½ cup almonds, thinly sliced
Bragg Liquid Aminos to taste
RealSalt to taste

Steam-fry onion and garlic in water, on low heat until softened. Add bean sprouts and stir until warm and slightly cooked. Add almonds. Add Bragg Liquid Aminos to taste. Season with RealSalt. Serve immediately.

Avocado Margarita

Contributed by Ashley Lisonbee

SERVES 6

½ small red onion, sliced
1 garlic clove, crushed
1 Tbs. olive oil
2 small tomatoes, diced
4 fresh basil leaves, torn into shreds
½ cup sprouts
2 Tbs. lemon juice
Salt and pepper to taste
3 avocados, halved and pitted

Combine all the ingredients in a bowl except for the avocado. Split avocado into two parts and take out the pit. Using the avocado halves as bowls, spoon the mixture into the center and serve.

Baked Eggplant Slices

Contributed by Linnette Webster
First place, pH Miracle 2004 Recipe Contest
Transitional Category

SERVES 4

1 eggplant, peeled and sliced into ⅜-inch slices
1 cup flour (any combination of amaranth or spelt berries, or sesame, flax, pumpkin, or sunflower seed)
1 tsp. salt
1 tsp. oregano
1 tsp. garlic powder
⅛ tsp. red pepper

Preheat the oven to 350 degrees F. Wash, peel, and slice eggplant into ⅜-inch slices. Stack slices, salting in between each slice (this removes bitterness). Let sit for 10 to 15 minutes, rinse and dry. Mix flour and seasonings. Coat each eggplant slice. Bake on oiled baking pan for 8 to 10 minutes on each side.

Baked Tofu

Contributed by Linnette Webster
First place, pH Miracle 2004 Recipe Contest
Transitional Category

SERVES 4–6

2 cartons tofu
¼ cup Bragg Liquid Aminos, or to taste
1¼ cups spelt flour
2 Tbs. onion powder
1 Tbs. parsley flakes
2 tsps. garlic powder
1 tsp. poultry seasoning
¼ tsp. red pepper

Preheat the oven to 350 degrees F. Cut tofu into ½-inch slices, drain. Sprinkle with Bragg Liquid Aminos to taste. Set aside. Mix dry ingredients together. Dip slices in dry mix to coat. Bake on oiled baking sheet 15 to 20 minutes. Turn, bake additional 15 minutes or until browned.

Variation:
• Substitute cracker crumbs for spelt flour for chunkier texture.

Brussels Sprouts Sauté

Contributed by Raye Haskell

SERVES 1

½ cup pure water
1 onion, diced
2 garlic cloves, diced

3 Brussels sprouts, shredded
Herbamare (A. Vogel) to taste

In water, sauté-steam-fry onion and garlic until softened. Add Brussels sprouts. Steam-fry until lightly cooked. Season with Herbamare. Serve warm.

Coconut Cream Fish Fillet

Contributed by Ashley Lisonbee

SERVES 2

Good side dish is steamed broccoli.

2 (1 lb.) fillets of fish

Sauce

1 (48 ml.) box of coconut cream
¾ tsp. RealSalt
¼ tsp. pepper or cayenne or Zip
½ lemon, juiced

Marinate fish in sauce for 2 hours in the refrigerator. Cook the fish on low-medium heat slowly in the sauce, flipping over for 1 to 3 minutes to let the sauce flavor the fish.

Deliciously Scrumptious Happy Salmon Burgers

Contributed by Myra Marvez Corbett
Second place, pH Miracle 2004 Recipe Contest
Transitional Category

SERVES 12–15

Why are they called happy salmon burgers? Because the salmon are still swimming in the ocean!

3 cups almonds, soaked at least 24 hours
2 cups carrot pulp, through Green Star machine
6–8 celery sticks, pulp
RealSalt to taste
2 tsps. ground dulse to taste
2 tsps. ground kelp to taste
1 red onion, chopped
Dash of powdered ginger (optional)

Use Green Star juice machine to press plumped almonds into pulp. Press and gather the pulp from the carrots and celery. Place into mixing bowl. Add remaining ingredients to the bowl. Mix well, adjusting seasonings to taste. Prepare dehydrator. Form mixture into patties and place on teflex sheets. Dehydrate for 5 to 6 hours. Patties can also be eaten raw.

Egg Rolls

Contributed by Linnette Webster
First place, pH Miracle 2004 Recipe Contest
Transitional Category

MAKES 12 ROLLS

3 cups cabbage
1 can bamboo shoots
1 can water chestnuts
4 green onions
2 Tbs. Bragg Liquid Aminos
1 tsp. five spice powder
2 tsps. salt
$^1/_{16}$ tsp. white stevia powder
Egg roll wrappers or sprouted wheat tortilla

Preheat the oven to 350 degrees F. In food processor grate cabbage. Place in mixing bowl. Pulse-chop bamboo shoots, water chestnuts, and green onions. Add to cabbage and mix. In a small mixing bowl, mix Bragg Liquid Aminos with seasonings and stevia. Pour over vegetables and mix thoroughly. Place ¼ cup vegetable mix in each egg roll skin. Fold one corner over filling and overlap the two opposite corners. Moisten the fourth corner with water and fold over to make a roll. Place on baking sheet, then brush with olive oil. Bake 15 to 20 minutes until browned. Serve with Hot Mustard (recipe follows), if desired.

Hot Mustard

3 Tbs. dry mustard
2 Tbs. water
1 Tbs. Bragg Liquid Aminos

Mix until smooth.

Esther's Hearty Sprouted Lentil Burgers

Contributed by Esther Andreas
Third place, pH Miracle 2004 Recipe Contest
Alkalizing Category

MAKES 2–3 DOZEN

A day ahead

2 cups lentils
½ cup sesame seeds or hemp
1 cup sunflower seeds
1 cup almonds

Soak all ingredients for 8 hours and then sprout for 4 hours. Chop finely in food processor and pour into a large bowl.

1½ cups onion
1 cup red bell pepper
6 garlic cloves
1 cup fresh basil
1 Tbs. lemon juice
½ tsp. Celtic Salt or RealSalt to taste
2 Tbs. fresh jalapeño pepper to taste
½ cup finely ground flaxseeds

Add to sprouted seeds and almond mixture, mix well. Make patties with ¼ cup scoop of mixture. Dehydrate on Teflex sheets for 3 hours at 115 degrees F. Turn over and remove Teflex sheets. Dehydrate for additional 3 hours. Burgers will keep in refrigerator for 1 week.

Esther's Spanish Quinoa

Contributed by Esther Andreas
Third place, pH Miracle 2004 Recipe Contest
Alkalizing Category

SERVES 6–8

1–1½ cups thinly sliced onion
2 Tbs. oil or 3 Tbs. water
1 red pepper, diced
1 orange pepper, diced
1 tsp. paprika
1 Tbs. minced garlic
1 tsp. RealSalt
3 cups fresh tomato juice or 3 cups blended fresh or frozen
    tomatoes
Cayenne pepper to taste
2 cups soaked and sprouted quinoa
2 small fresh tomatoes, chopped
1 green onion
3 Tbs. fresh cilantro

The day before, or 4 to 6 hours before, rinse and soak quinoa until just sprouted. Sauté or steam-fry, on low heat, onions in oil or water for 3 minutes. Add peppers, paprika, garlic, salt, 3 cups of the blended tomatoes (or juice), cayenne, and quinoa. Stir well. Bring to a gentle boil for 5 minutes. Take off heat and let sit for 30 minutes. Just before serving, fold in the freshly chopped tomato, green onion, and cilantro.

Garlic Cauliflower "Potatoes"

Contributed by Denise Finocchio
First place, pH Miracle 2004 Recipe Contest
Transitional Category

SERVES 3–4

1 head of cauliflower
1 tsp. garlic powder or to taste
½ tsp. RealSalt
½ tsp. basil, fresh or dried
1–3 Tbs. olive oil

Steam cauliflower with garlic powder, RealSalt, and basil. In food processor, pulse-chop cauliflower and seasonings until smooth as mashed "potatoes." Add olive oil. Blend.

Lettuce/Cabbage Wraps

Contributed by Ashley Lisonbee

SERVES 8–10

1 head of cabbage
1 carrot, cut into matchsticks
2 celery stalks, cut into matchsticks
1 cucumber, cut into matchsticks
2 cups bean sprouts
½ pkg. of buckwheat soba noodles

Hot Sweet Sauce

½ cup coconut milk
2 Tbs. olive oil

½ tsp. salt
½ tsp. Zip (Spice Hunter)
¼ tsp. crushed red pepper
½ tsp. ground mustard
Dash of stevia

Wash 8 to 10 cabbage leaves. Set aside. Cut carrot, celery, and cucumber into matchstick pieces. Rinse bean sprouts. Prepare soba noodles as directed on package, boiling in water for 5 to 8 minutes. Mix sauce ingredients in a bowl with a fork. To assemble each wrap, place matchstick veggies in the center of the cabbage leaf, along with a small spoonful of soba noodles. Roll cabbage leaf until it hugs the veggies and noodles. Dip in sauce for flavor or add 1 to 2 tsps. of sauce in each cabbage roll.

Mexican Stack Up with Tofu Sausage

Donated by Victoria's Gourmet—Victoria Frerichs
Professional Award, pH Miracle 2004 Recipe Contest

EACH TOSTADA SERVES 1

Build a tostada directly on plate (or use sprouted tortilla). Start with your favorite beans. Add nutrition and color by layering onions, peppers, and shredded veggies. Top with Tofu Sausage (recipe follows) and seasonings.

Tofu Sausage

Packaged extra-firm tofu
Oil
To taste: sage, salt, red pepper flakes (or cayenne), marjoram,
   thyme, Zip

Press tofu in glass pan as follows: Drain tofu. Layer tofu slice, four layers of paper towels, tofu slice, paper towel, paper plate, cans, or books to add weight. Leave overnight in fridge. Crumble pressed tofu. Stir-fry in neutral oil until starts to be crisp. Add sage, salt, red pepper flakes (or cayenne), marjoram, thyme, and Zip.

Michael's Pizza Tortilla

Contributed by Michael Steadman
Second place, pH Miracle 2004 Recipe Contest
Transitional Category

SERVES 1

1 sprouted tortilla
Sun-Dried Tomato Spread (page 285)
Vegetables of choice: red, yellow, orange, or green bell pepper,
celery, onion, tomato, spinach (fresh or roasted)
Seasonings: oregano and basil
Avocado, sliced

Toast tortilla in the oven on low heat or in the dehydrator overnight. Spread sun-dried tomato spread on tortilla. Chop vegetables. Load vegetables on tortilla. Top with seasonings to taste. Add avocado. Serve warm or cold.

Mixed Veggie Lentils

Contributed by Ashley Lisonbee

SERVES 4–6

1 cup green lentils
4 Tbs. olive oil or grapeseed oil
2 garlic cloves, crushed
1 Tbs. lime or lemon juice

1 small red onion, cut into eighths
1 yellow bell pepper
1 red bell pepper
½ cup green beans, halved
½ cup vegetable broth
Dash of crushed red pepper
Salt and Zip (Spice Hunter) to taste
Dash of stevia

Soak lentils in a large pan of cold water for 25 minutes. Bring to a boil, reduce heat, and simmer for 10 minutes on low, drain thoroughly. Add 1 Tbs. of the olive or grapeseed oil, 1 of the garlic cloves, and lime juice to lentils and mix well. Set aside. Heat remaining olive or grapeseed oil in a pan and stir-fry the remaining garlic lightly. Add the onion, bell peppers, and green beans. Stir-fry for 4 to 5 minutes. Add the vegetable broth to the pan and simmer for 10 minutes on medium-low heat. Add lentils to veggies and add pepper, salt, Zip, and a dash of stevia to taste.

Variations:
- Use different veggies like zucchini, carrots, and snow peas, or for a creamier version add 2 Tbs. of coconut cream.
- For a raw dish, sprout the lentils and add into mixed veggies and lightly warm.

Purple Edamame Stir-Fry

Contributed by Ashley Lisonbee

SERVES 4

This is a great side dish!

7 oz. tofu, extra firm
1 Tbs. grapeseed oil
2 Tbs. sesame seeds
2 cups purple cabbage, shredded
1 cup edamame beans
1½ Tbs. fresh lemon juice
¾ tsp. RealSalt
¼ tsp. crushed red pepper
Dash of stevia

Cut tofu into ½-inch slices. In a pan add oil and sliced tofu. Warm on medium heat until lightly toasted. Add sesame seeds and toast with tofu for 2 minutes. Add cabbage and edamame and warm for additional 5 minutes. Add lemon juice, spices, and stevia. Stir and serve warm.

Quinoa Tabbouleh

Contributed by Ashley Lisonbee

SERVES 6

1 cup quinoa
1 cup water
½ cup fresh lemon juice
⅓ cup olive oil
1 cup red onion
4 garlic cloves
1 cup Italian parsley, coarsely chopped

Salt and Zip (Spice Hunter) to taste
4 plum tomatoes, cut in ½-inch pieces
1 English cucumber, cut into ½-inch pieces

Rinse quinoa. Steam with water until all water is absorbed (25 to 30 minutes). Cool in mixing bowl. Add the lemon juice and oil. In food processor, finely chop onion and garlic. Add to quinoa with parsley, salt, and Zip. Mix well. Add tomatoes and cucumbers and chill in refrigerator for 30 minutes. Serve cold.

Roasted Cajun Vegetables

Contributed by Ashley Lisonbee

SERVES 2–4

1 yam
3 carrots
½ red onion
2 zucchini
1 red bell pepper
1 green bell pepper
3 Tbs. olive oil
½ lime, juiced

Cajun Spice

2 tsps. paprika
1 tsp. cumin
1 tsp. coriander
1 tsp. black pepper (optional)
½–1 tsp. chili powder

Preheat the oven to 450 degrees F. Chop all veggies into bite-sized pieces. Put oil, lime juice, Cajun spices, and chopped vegetables into a gallon-size Ziploc bag. Toss veggies in the spice until well covered.

Empty veggies onto a foil-covered cookie sheet. Spread out so they cover the pan evenly. Bake for 15 to 20 minutes. Reduce heat to 375 degrees F and bake for another 15 minutes until veggies are tender.

Seed Pancakes with Whipped Topping

Contributed by Linnette Webster
First place, pH Miracle 2004 Recipe Contest
Transitional Category

SERVES 2

Flour Mix

¼ cup raw pumpkin seeds
¼ cup raw sunflower seeds
¼ cup raw sesame seeds
½ cup raw flaxseeds

Pancake Mix

1 cup seed flour
1 cup millet or spelt flour or combination of quinoa, amaranth, buckwheat, bean flour
1½ tsps. baking soda
1 tsp. RealSalt
$^1/_{16}$ tsp. stevia
Soymilk, unsweetened
Olive oil

For Flour Mix: Measure out seeds and mix together. In coffee grinder, grind seeds into flour in ⅓ cup batches. Measure 1 cup for seed pancakes. Reserve rest for other recipes (store in airtight container in refrigerator). For Pancake Mix: Mix dry ingredients until just blended. Add just enough soymilk to achieve thin batter (batter thickens after sitting a couple of minutes). Heat skillet, oil pan, pour thin layer of batter. Flip pancakes when bubbles rise. Serve with Whipped Topping (recipe follows).

Variation:
• ***Buckwheat Pancakes.*** Use 2 cups buckwheat flour (grind raw buckwheat kernels), 1½ tsps. soda, 1 tsp. salt, ¹/₁₆ tsp. stevia powder (optional), water or soymilk.
• ***Anything Pancakes.*** Use any combination of flours (seed, nut, grain, bean) in same proportions as buckwheat mix.

Whipped Topping

Contributed by Linnette Webster
First place, pH Miracle 2004 Recipe Contest
Transitional Category

MAKES 1 CUP

½ carton silken (soft) tofu
⅓ cup coconut milk (Thai Kitchen)
1–2 tsps. vanilla, nonalcohol (Frontier)
⅛ tsp. white stevia powder
1 Tbs. lemon juice

In food processor, blend ingredients until smooth and creamy.

Shanghai Pedro

Contributed by Maraline Krey
First place, pH Miracle 2004 Recipe Contest
Alkalizing Category

SERVES 4 (8 LETTUCE WRAPS OR 4 TORTILLA WRAPS)

8 lettuce leaves, such as Boston lettuce

Puree Sauce

1 red bell pepper
1½ carrots
2–3 Tbs. ginger, pureed
1 Tbs. garlic, pureed
1½ Tbs. Bragg Liquid Aminos
Stevia to taste

3 veggie burgers
Salt and pepper to taste
¼ cup onion
1½ cups prepared black beans
celery
carrot
red onion

Optional Basmati Rice

2 cups vegetable broth
2 Tbs. green onion, minced
1 cup basmati rice

Vegetables

⅓ cup celery, diced in ½-inch pieces
⅓ cup carrots, diced in ¼-inch pieces
⅓ cup broccoli, diced in ¼-inch pieces
½ cup red cabbage, shredded
⅓ cup sprouts

Wash lettuce leaves and while wet, lay each leaf on a paper towel. Press your thumb on the vein of the leaf to flatten vein, then roll into a tube (each leaf tube making a "taco shell"). Refrigerate.

Tip: If using a tortilla, place a dry lettuce leaf into the tortilla. Roll (this will prevent tortilla from breaking up and will add crunch). Refrigerate. In food processor, puree sauce ingredients. Pan-sear veggie burgers with seasonings and onion. Cut burgers into ½-inch chunks and return to pan. Add beans. Add pureed sauce, stir and remove from heat. Unroll lettuce "taco shells," fill each with heated veggie burger/bean mixture. Top with rice and diced vegetables.

Shredded Zucchini

Contributed by Raye Haskell

SERVES 4

1 bunch green onions (heads and greens), chopped
3 garlic cloves, chopped
2 Tbs. olive oil
4 large zucchini, chopped
2 Tbs. almonds, soaked and sliced
Herbamare (A. Vogel) to taste

Sauté onions and garlic in olive oil on low heat until slightly tender. Add zucchini and stir into mixture. Warm until zucchini begins to soften. Add almonds and toss. Season with Herbamare to taste.

Simply Alkalarian

Quick and Easy Make to Taste
Contributed by Maraline Krey
First place, pH Miracle 2004 Recipe Contest
Alkalizing Category
This array of tasty shortcuts and tasty tidbits are for Alkalarians who have little time but very big appetites for the Alkalarian lifestyle. Says Maraline: "Let's not 'substitute,' but let us 'replace' with better tasting, better for you, and, most important, better results!"

Simple Meals

Layer raw with cooked, or create bowls.
Rice/Pasta: Prepare enough rice for two meals.

Basmati Rice Options

Cooking Liquid Variations:
  • Soup base
  • Almond milk pureed with 3 or 4 strands of saffron
  • Coconut milk pureed with cinnamon
  • Choice of spices

Quinoa or Spinach Pasta Options
Toss cooked/drained pasta in good oils (i.e., avocado, extra-virgin olive oil, coconut oil, and dash of RealSalt).
Add choice of raw tomato, herbs, veggies, avocado, etc.
Prepare rice or pasta, place in bowls or on plate (or over raw spinach) and use your choice from Simple Sauces.

Sample Layered Plate
Base: Raw spinach or salad greens tossed with equal parts lime and good oil with RealSalt. Place on plate.
Add choice of rice or pasta.
Top with one or more of the following:
Fresh veggies, raw, lightly steamed, or stir-fried
Grilled cold water/wild fish brushed with avocado oil and spices, or steamed
Cover with any Simple Sauce of choice.

Spaghetti Squash with Pumpkin Seed Pesto

Contributed by Lisa El-Kerdi
Best in Show, pH Miracle 2004 Recipe Contest

SERVES 4–6

This versatile dish may be served as a side dish, main course, or salad. Freeze pesto in ice cube trays and remove for soups, stews, or individual servings. An addition of fresh arugula makes an interesting addition.

1 spaghetti squash, baked
Pumpkin Seed Pesto (recipe follows)

Preheat the oven to 350 degrees F. Bake squash until it yields slightly to pressure, but still is firm, approximately 30 to 45 minutes. Remove seeds and pull spaghetti strands with fork. Toss with pesto and serve.

Pumpkin Seed Pesto

3 cloves garlic
1 tsp. RealSalt
Black pepper, freshly ground
2 cups fresh basil leaves
1 cup pumpkin seeds
1 cup olive oil

Combine garlic, salt, and pepper in food processor and chop finely. Add basil leaves and pumpkin seeds. Blend until ground. With motor running, slowly add olive oil and blend until well combined.

Variations:
- Add steamed or raw vegetables, sun-dried tomatoes, or artichoke hearts to basic recipe.

Spelt Flour Tortillas

Contributed by Karen Ellis
Honorable Mention, pH Miracle 2004 Recipe Contest

2 cups spelt flour
1 cup water
¼ cup olive oil
½ tsp. RealSalt or sea salt
Any other seasonings of choice

Form ingredients into large ball and knead until smooth on a pastry board covered with spelt flour. Pull off 2-inch ball and roll out flat into round tortilla shape. Bake on pizza grill or large frying pan until both sides are bubbly and brown. Serve with refried beans, avocado, tomatoes, fresh salsa, and so forth.

Spelt/Quinoa Manicotti Shells with Marinara Sauce

Contributed by Denise Finocchio
First place, pH Miracle 2004 Recipe Contest
Transitional Category

SERVES 6 (18 SHELLS)

Shells

1¼ cups quinoa flour
1¼ cups spelt flour
4½ tsps. egg replacer (Ener G)
RealSalt
2 cups pure water
Oil for frying

Filling

1 package firm tofu
½ cup vegetable parmesan cheese
1 garlic clove, minced
½ cup parsley, fresh minced
½ cup basil, fresh minced

Preheat the oven to 350 degrees F. For the Shells: Combine all ingredients except oil. Batter should be the consistency of thin pancake or crepe mix. Oil an electric skillet. Ladle out 2 Tbs. batter for a thin pancake. Flip when slightly browned. Stack until needed. For the Filling: In food processor blend first three ingredients until smooth and creamy. Add next two ingredients and pulse a few times to mix in. Prepare a 9 × 9-inch pan with healthy oil. Cover bottom of pan with freshly made marinara sauce (recipe follows). Place 2 Tbs. of filling in the middle of the pancake. Roll flap under the cheese. Place flip side down in pan. When all are assembled, cover with marina sauce and sprinkle with vegetable parmesan cheese. Cover with tinfoil and bake for 30 minutes. Uncover, top with soy mozzarella, and bake another 20 minutes. Serve on plate, and top with fresh marinara sauce and vegetable parmesan cheese.

Variations:
• Add veggies like squash, zucchini, carrots, and broccoli.

Marinara Sauce

Contributed by Denise Finocchio
First place, pH Miracle 2004 Recipe Contest
Transitional Category

MAKES 2–3 CUPS

12 sun-dried tomatoes, soaked 1 hour
1 onion, minced
4 garlic cloves, minced
⅓ cup basil, chopped
1 large can plum tomatoes with basil, and juices
10 oz. pure water
RealSalt to taste

In food processor, puree sun-dried tomatoes. In a large saucepan, sauté onions and garlic in oil and add basil. Add sun-dried tomato puree to onions and garlic. Sauté for additional 3 minutes to blend flavors. Add canned plum tomatoes and water to pan. Cook on medium heat for 10 minutes. Reduce heat to low, simmering additional 30 minutes to 1 hour. Add salt to taste.

Variation:
  • Use fresh plum tomatoes instead of canned. Add only 1 cup of water. Increase water to thin sauce if desired.

Spicy Coconut Crusted Salmon with Roasted Garlic and Sun-Dried Tomato Cream Sauce

Contributed by Jana McCutcheon
Honorable Mention, pH Miracle 2004 Recipe Contest

SERVES 6

1½ cups fresh coconut, finely shredded
2 Tbs. dried parsley
2 Tbs. dried oregano
3 tsps. paprika
2 Tbs. granulated garlic
1 tsp. RealSalt
1 tsp. black pepper (optional)
½ tsp. cayenne or to taste
¼ cup olive oil
6 (3 oz.) salmon fillets

Preheat the oven to 350 degrees F. Spread coconut in a 9 × 13-inch baking dish and toast until dry and golden, about 10 minutes. Remove from oven, add spices, stirring to combine. Increase oven temperature to 400 degrees F. Line broiler pan with foil and brush with olive oil. Brush both sides of each salmon piece with olive oil and roll in coconut mixture to coat. Bake for 15 to 20 minutes, or until fish flakes easily. Top with Roasted Garlic and Sun-Dried Tomato Cream Sauce (recipe follows).

Roasted Garlic and Sun-Dried Tomato Cream Sauce

MAKES 2 CUPS

1 tsp. granulated garlic
6–8 sun-dried tomatoes, finely chopped
2 cups vegetable broth
2 cups fresh almond milk
1 garlic bulb, roasted
1 tsp. onion powder
1 tsp. RealSalt
½–1 tsp. black pepper (optional)

In food processor pulse-chop roasted garlic and sun-dried tomatoes together. Combine all ingredients into a saucepan over medium heat. Bring to a gentle boil, stirring often, reducing mixture until thick, about 15 to 20 minutes. Serving suggestions: Pour over fish, pastas, or vegetables.

Stacks

Contributed by Linnette Webster
First place, pH Miracle 2004 Recipe Contest
Transitional Category

Stacks are easy, layered meals, akin to the tostada. They often start with a warm, grounding grain or legume and are topped with fresh vegetables and low-sugar fruits or nuts. End with olive oil and lemon juice, Bragg Liquid Aminos, or an alternative sauce. Beginning a stack with a vegetable works too. The nice thing about a stack is it adapts to whatever is in your refrigerator. Here are some examples to get you started:

• Quinoa, steamed broccoli, tomatoes, red onion, radishes, chopped Brazil nuts

- Brown rice, chopped avocado, soaked almonds (or sunflower, sesame, pumpkin seeds), chopped zucchini, and green onions
- Cooked lentils, steam-fried onions and garlic, fresh or steamed kale
- Steamed mustard greens (or other greens), sautéed onions, guacamole
- Raw cooked buckwheat, freeze-dried coconut, soaked almonds, finely shredded cabbage, chopped broccoli, thinly sliced radishes, cherry tomatoes
- Sprouted wheat tortilla crisped in skillet in olive oil, refried pinto beans, spinach, lettuce, sprouted alfalfa, fresh salsa
- Sprouted buckwheat, grated fresh coconut, stevia, unsweetened soymilk, sprouted seeds—almost breakfast cereal!
- Cooked millet, steamed Brussels sprouts, and onions
- Steamed broccoli, sunflower seeds, diced red bell pepper, radishes
- Cooked quinoa, raw grated carrot, chopped broccoli, cauliflower, onion, cabbage, almonds, and avocado, mixed and warmed in skillet

Steamed Fish and Greens in Coconut Water

SERVES 4

1 lb. fresh salmon, trout, or red snapper fillets, with skin on
RealSalt to taste
Garlic Herb Bread Seasoning (Spice Hunter)
1 Tbs. fresh ginger, cut in thin slices or grated
1 cup yellow chives
½ cup green chives
4 cups fresh kale
2 Tbs. Bragg Liquid Aminos
1 young Thai coconut water, cracked and water drained
½ cup cilantro

In a nonstick fry pan, lay the fish, skin side down, and steam-fry with the lid on until the fish is cooked through but also moist. Halfway through, remove the lid and sprinkle fish with RealSalt and Garlic Herb Bread Seasoning. When the fish flakes easily, remove carefully to a plate and set aside. Take the skin off the fish and discard, but leave any oils from the fish in the pan. Place the thinly sliced ginger in the oiled pan and cook until the ginger is browned. Add all other ingredients except cilantro and steam in the pan with the lid on until bright green and softened. Add the fish back to pan, topping with cilantro. Steam 1 or 2 more minutes before serving.

Stir-Fry: UN-Cashew Chicken

Contributed by Kelley Anclien
Second place, pH Miracle 2004 Recipe Contest
Alkalizing Category

SERVES 4

2 cups brown rice, cooked
2 Tbs. olive oil
RealSalt to taste
3 Tbs. grapeseed oil
Onion, minced
Garlic, minced
Celery, diced
7 baby carrots, diced circles
½ green bell pepper, chopped
½ cup broccoli, chopped
Szechwan Seasoning (Spice Hunter)
⅛ tsp. red pepper flakes
1 lemon, juiced
Bragg Liquid Aminos to taste
½–1 cup Marcona Almonds (Mitica)

Cook brown rice. Add olive oil, salt to taste. Coat pan with 1 Tbs. of the grapeseed oil, add vegetables, stir-fry on low. Add remaining 2 Tbs. of the grapeseed oil, sprinkle vegetables with Szechwan Seasoning and red pepper flakes. Stir in lemon juice. Stir-fry 3 to 5 minutes, mixing seasonings and oil to coat vegetables thoroughly. Remove from heat, add Bragg Liquid Aminos. Top with almonds.

Summer Vegetable Strata

Contributed by Lisa El-Kerdi
Best in Show, pH Miracle 2004 Recipe Contest

SERVES 12–16

2 large Vidalia onions
8 yellow squash
8 zucchini
2 large or 4 small eggplants
2 green bell peppers
4 lbs. tomatoes
RealSalt
Italian seasoning
Olive oil
Crushed red pepper

Preheat the oven to 425 degrees F. Coat sides and bottom of deep rectangular roasting pan with olive oil. Slice onions and place at bottom of pan. Slice squash and other vegetables about $3/16$-inch thick as you layer into pan in order above. Reserve some squash and zucchini to slice in lengthwise strips for topping. Every other layer, sprinkle lightly with salt and seasoning (not red pepper) and drizzle with olive oil. Use thin slices of tomato for inner layer, saving most of the tomatoes for the next-to-last layer. After completing first layer, repeat using focus vegetables. Cover with most of the tomatoes. Sprinkle with salt, seasoning, and red pepper and drizzle with olive oil. Bake 20 minutes.

Top

For the top layer, cut an equal amount of zucchini and yellow squash in half crosswise. Slice in thin lengthwise slices. Remove pan from oven and place alternating strips of yellow squash and zucchini first down one side of the pan then repeating on the other. If you don't have enough squash to cover top, make open-lattice-work design. Brush with olive oil and return to oven until all vegetables are tender, approximately 20 minutes. Remove from oven. Allow to cool for 15 minutes to set. Cut into squares and remove from pan with spatula.

Tofu Chow Mien

Contributed by Linnette Webster
First place, pH Miracle 2004 Recipe Contest
Transitional Category

SERVES 4–6

2 cartons tofu
2–3 tsps. Bragg Liquid Aminos
3 onions, cut in lengthwise strips
4 garlic cloves, minced
1 tsp. gingerroot, grated
6 celery stalks, thinly sliced
2 carrots, thinly sliced
1 cup pure water
1 Tbs. RealSalt
1 can bean sprouts, or 1½ cups fresh
1 can water chestnuts, sliced
1 can bamboo shoots
1 Tbs. arrowroot powder
¼ cup pure water

Freeze container of tofu (this makes tofu chewier, more meat-like). Preheat the oven to 400 degrees F. Thaw tofu before preparation and drain. Squeeze out water, cut into ½-inch cubes. Sprinkle with Bragg Liquid Aminos, spread cubes on oiled baking pan, and bake for 30 minutes until lightly brown. Sauté onions, garlic, and gingerroot until lightly transparent. Add celery, carrots, water, and salt to steam-fry for 2 minutes. Add, just to warm, bean sprouts, bamboo shoots, and water chestnuts. Mix together arrowroot powder and ¼ cup water. Add to vegetables to thicken broth. Add tofu cube and warm slightly. Serve over brown rice or quinoa.

Turkish Moussaka (Eggplant Casserole)

Contributed by Linnette Webster
First place, pH Miracle 2004 Recipe Contest
Transitional Category

SERVES 4

1–2 cartons silken tofu, soft
Salt
2 eggplants
3 cups Sneaky Tomato Sauce (recipe follows)

Sneaky Tomato Sauce

SERVES 8

1 medium onion
1 medium green pepper
2 carrots
2 celery stalks
3 large (5 small) tomatoes
½ cup fresh parsley, chopped
3 garlic cloves, minced
1 tsp. basil, fresh minced or dried
½ tsp. oregano
1 (16-oz.) can tomato sauce
1 (6-oz.) can tomato paste
¼ cup olive oil

Chop onion and green pepper in food processor and steam-fry until almost tender. Chop carrots and celery in processor and add to the onions and peppers; steam-fry a few more minutes. In a blender, combine tomatoes, half the vegetable mixture, parsley, garlic, basil, and oregano. Pour into a large saucepan or skillet. Using same blender, mix tomato sauce, remaining vegetable mixture, tomato paste, and olive oil. Add to saucepan, and heat to serve.

Topping

6 Tbs. spelt flour
¼ cup olive oil
2 cups soymilk, unsweetened
1 tsp. RealSalt
1 garlic clove, minced
2 Tbs. tahini

Bread Crumb Finale

3 slices yeast-free millet bread, cubed
2 Tbs. olive oil
1 tsp. RealSalt

Freeze container of tofu (this makes tofu chewier, more meat-like). Preheat the oven to 350 degrees F. Thaw tofu before preparation and cut tofu into ⅜-inch cubes. Lightly salt and bake in oiled baking pan 15 minutes, turn cubes, bake additional 15 minutes. Wash, peel, and slice eggplant into ⅜-inch slices. Stack slices, salting in between each slice. (This removes bitterness.) Let sit for 15 to 20 minutes, rinse, and dry. Rinse slices and steam until tender, 10 minutes. Layer tomato sauce, eggplant slices, tofu cubes, ending with a sauce layer. Prepare "topping" in a skillet, on medium heat. Whisk together spelt flour and olive oil. Add soymilk and seasonings and cook until thickened. Spread over top layers of tomato sauce, eggplant, and tofu slices. Mix "bread crumb finale" ingredients in a bowl. Spread mixture on top of casserole. Bake for 15 minutes to warm and brown crumb topping.

Veggie Jambalaya

Contributed by Ashley Lisonbee

SERVES 6

1 cup brown rice
2 Tbs. olive oil
1 red onion, cut into eighths
2 garlic cloves, crushed
1 green bell pepper, diced
1 red bell pepper, diced
1 eggplant, diced
½ cup green peas
1 cup broccoli florets cut into small pieces
⅔ cup vegetable broth
8 oz. fresh vine ripe tomatoes, diced
1 tsp. organic tomato paste
½ tsp. cumin
½ tsp. paprika
½ tsp. chili powder
1 tsp. salt
½ tsp. Zip (Spice Hunter)

Cook rice with 2 cups of water in large pan for 20 minutes or until soft and water is absorbed. Set aside. Heat oil in skillet and warm onion and garlic for 3 minutes. Add the peppers, eggplant, peas, and broccoli stirring occasionally additional 3 minutes. Stir in vegetable broth, tomatoes, tomato paste, and seasonings. Adjust seasonings to taste, mix well. Warm for 15 minutes. Stir brown rice into vegetables and serve warm.

Wild Asian Salmon

Contributed by Maraline Krey
First place, pH Miracle 2004 Recipe Contest
Alkalizing Category

SERVES 4

Pesto

½ Tbs. ginger
3 garlic cloves
¼ cup cilantro
¼ mint
¼ cup parsley
3–4 limes, juiced
1 Tbs. coconut oil
1 tsp. sesame oil
1 tsp. Bragg Liquid Aminos
RealSalt to taste

Salmon

4 salmon fillets, wild catch

Rice

1 Tbsp avocado oil
1 Tbs. onion, minced
1 cup basmati rice
1 cup vegetable broth
1 cup coconut milk

Salad

½ lime, juiced
¼ cup avocado oil
RealSalt to taste
Pepper to taste
2 cups baby spinach

Garnish

Sesame seeds
Sprigs of mint and cilantro

For Pesto: In food processor, blend ingredients until smooth. Prepare salmon. Cut into 8 pieces, rinse and pat dry. Arrange in single layer on oil-rubbed baking sheet. Brush all sides of fillets with pesto. Cover and refrigerate until ready to pan-sear. Oil a nonstick searing pan. Spritz salmon with oil, pan-sear about 2 or 3 minutes on each side. For the rice: Heat oil in pan and add onion. Cook for 2 minutes. Add rice, broth, and milk, reduce heat, cover for 45 minutes. For the salad: Juice lime into a dish, add oil, and whisk in salt and pepper. Toss baby spinach leaves until coated. *Presentation:* Layer half of the plate with spinach salad. Place 2 salmon pieces on top, garnish with sesame seeds. Serve with rice alongside and garnish with sesame seeds, mint, and cilantro.

SNACKS/DESSERTS

Almost Apple Pie

Contributed by Debra Jenkins
Second place, pH Miracle 2004 Recipe Contest
Alkalizing Category

MAKES 1 (8-INCH) PIE

4 cups jicama, grated
¼ cup almond meal, fresh or Bob's Red Mill
¼ tsp. RealSalt
2 tsps. nutmeg
4 tsps. cinnamon
½ tsp cloves, ground
1 cup freeze-dried coconut flakes (Wilderness Family Naturals preferred)
4 tsps. psyllium flakes
¼ cup coconut oil, melted (Wilderness Family Naturals preferred)
2 Tbs. vanilla flavoring, alcohol-free (Frontier)
2 tsps. lemon flavoring, alcohol-free (Frontier)
1½ cups almond milk (fresh preferred)

Set aside grated jicama. Mix in a bowl almond meal, salt, nutmeg, cinnamon, cloves, coconut flakes, and psyllium flakes. Set aside. Melt together coconut oil, flavorings, and almond milk. Mix melted ingredients with dry ingredients. Add grated jicama and fold together until thoroughly moistened. Place in pie dish, pat to flatten, and cool in refrigerator for 1 hour. Ready to serve.

Variations:
- Coconut Meal Pie Crust (page 329) is a great crust for this pie.
- Substitute agar flakes (4 tsps.) for psyllium flakes.

- Substitute water for almond milk during cleanse. Or for rich pie, use coconut cream instead of almond milk.
- Substitute fresh lemon juice only if water is used for almond milk.
- Top with coconut cream or spread (Wilderness Family Naturals).

Barbeque Buffalo Chips

Serves 4–6

These little miniburgers have a grain-like texture because you just soak the seeds and nuts an hour before using. When you process them, leave the mixture a little coarse—very hearty and filling. Break up over a salad or dehydrate into crackers. Or use the batter (process until smoother) uncooked as a rich paté or spread.

2 cups fresh-soaked pecans (rinse and soak 1 hour)
1 cup fresh-soaked sunflower seeds (rinse and soak 1 hour)
¼ cup fresh-soaked pumpkin seeds (rinse and soak 1 hour)
½ large Flax Cracker (raw wheat-free crusts, Mauk Family Farms): a blend of gold and brown flaxseeds, sesame seeds, and sunflower seeds, with garlic, onion, celery seed, red bell pepper, parsley, sea salt, and pepper, dehydrated at 105 degrees.
1 Tbs. of Cowboy Barbeque Rub seasoning (Spice Hunter), more if you like a real barbeque kick
½–1 tsp. RealSalt or to taste

Soak all nuts and seeds for 1 hour and then rinse and drain. Into a Cuisinart food processor, place all ingredients and process until slightly coarse. Mold into small patties and pan-fry until golden on each side. Sprinkle more Cowboy Barbeque Rub on each side for color and more flavor. Serve hot off the pan.

Carrot "Apple" Cake

Contributed by Lisa El-Kerdi
Best in Show, pH Miracle 2004 Recipe Contest

2 pkgs. silken tofu
1¼ cups grapeseed oil
½ cup water (approximate)
3 cups grated carrots
1 cup finely chopped jicama
1 cup chopped walnuts or pecans
¾ to 1 cup unsweetened coconut flakes
2 Tbs. stevia
2 cups spelt flour, fresh ground if possible
2 tsps. baking soda
½ tsp. salt
3 tsps. cinnamon

Preheat the oven to 350 degrees F (375 F for high altitude). Grease a 9 × 13-inch pan or two 9-inch pans with coconut oil or line muffin tins with cupcake papers. Puree tofu. Cream tofu and oil. Add water, beating until mixture is smooth. Fold in next four ingredients. Sift dry ingredients together and add slowly. Mix cake until all is well blended. Bake approximately 1 hour or until toothpick inserted in cake comes out almost clean. Cool. Serve as is or frost with Coconut Crème (recipe follows). Keep refrigerated, particularly if frosted.

Variations: These 3 ingredients are for a spicier cake:
1 tsp. powdered ginger (optional)
¼ tsp. nutmeg (optional)
pinch cloves (optional)

Wedding Cake

Prepare layered cake, using graded circular pans and making several recipes as necessary. Frost cake with Coconut Crème (recipe follows). Sprinkle unsweetened coconut flakes over frosting. Refrigerate cake. Before serving, decorate with fresh organic flowers.

Coconut Crème

Contributed by Lisa El-Kerdi
Best in Show, pH Miracle 2004 Recipe Contest

MAKES ENOUGH TO FROST 1 (9-INCH) LAYER CAKE

1 pkg. silken tofu, soft
¼ cup coconut oil (Wilderness Family Farms preferred)
½ cup canned unsweetened coconut milk, or to desired consistency
½–1 tsp. white stevia (to taste)
2 tsps. alcohol-free vanilla
1 tsp. lime juice
1½ tsps. psyllium husk
Unsweetened coconut flakes (optional)

In food processor, blend all ingredients except psyllium husk. When smooth, correct seasonings and add psyllium husk, blending until completely incorporated. Serve as a topping or icing. This also makes a great meringue substitute! Add coconut flakes to crème or sprinkle on top, if desired.

Carrot Cake

Contributed by Linnette Webster
First place, pH Miracle 2004 Recipe Contest
Transitional Category

MAKES 1 (8 × 8-INCH) PAN

½ cup seed flour combination (2 Tbs. raw pumpkin seeds,
2 Tbs. raw sunflower seeds, 2 Tbs. sesame seeds,
4 Tbs. flaxseed)
1 cup spelt flour
½ cup amaranth flour (grind from seeds)
1½ tsps. baking soda
1 tsp. RealSalt
¼–½ tsp. white stevia powder
2 tsps. cinnamon
2 dashes nutmeg
1 cup minus 2 Tbs. soymilk, unsweetened
⅓ cup olive oil or coconut oil
1 tsp. lemon juice
½ tsp. vanilla, non-alcohol (Frontier)
2 cups carrots, finely grated

Preheat the oven to 350 degrees F. Grind seed for seed flour in coffee grinder in ⅓ cup batches. Combine dry ingredients and mix well. Combine liquid ingredients. Mix together dry and liquid ingredients just until blended. Fold in grated carrots. Pour into oiled 8 × 8-inch baking pan. Bake for 20 minutes. Serve with Whipped Topping (page 305).

Coconut Meal Pie Crust

Contributed by Debra Jenkins
Second place, pH Miracle 2004 Recipe Contest
Alkalizing Category

MAKES 1 (8-INCH) PIE

¾ cup almond meal
¼ cup flax meal
2 Tbs. spelt flour (can be omitted, if preferred)
½ plus 1 cup freeze-dried coconut flakes (Wilderness Family Naturals)
½ tsp. RealSalt
¼ tsp. agar flakes
3 Tbs. coconut oil (Wilderness Family Naturals)
2 Tbs. water

Mix dry ingredients. Melt coconut oil and add to dry ingredients. Add water. Drop into a pie plate and pat crust into place. Fill with favorite filling.

Colossal Coconut Crust and Pie

Contributed by Linda Broadhead
Third place, pH Miracle 2004 Recipe Contest
Transitional Category

SERVES 6–8

Crust

1 cup pine nuts
1 cup almonds, soaked
¼ cup shredded coconut flakes
⅛ tsp. RealSalt
2 Tbs. coconut oil

Filling

1 can Thai coconut milk or ½ young coconut meat plus ½–1 cup
    water
½ avocado
4 drops flavoring of choice, peppermint, lemon, etc.
½–1 tsp. SlimSweet, stevia
1 tsp. alcohol-free vanilla flavoring
⅛ tsp. RealSalt
½ tsp. agar flakes, to thicken

For the crust: Chop crust ingredients in a food processor.
Pat onto pie plate. For the filling: In food processor, blend all filling ingredients until smooth. Pour into pie crust. Refrigerate to
thicken.

Dill Toasties

Contributed by Lisa El-Kerdi
Best in Show, pH Miracle 2004 Recipe Contest

SERVES 16–20

1 package Ezekial Sprouted Grain Tortillas
Olive oil
Dried dill weed (or other favorite seasonings)
Sesame seeds
RealSalt

Preheat the oven to 300 degrees F. Brush tortillas with olive oil.
Sprinkle with herbs, seeds, and salt. Stack tortillas and slice into 8
wedges (halves, quarters, eighths). Bake on cookie sheet for 12 to 15
minutes, until light golden and crisp.

Michael's Bars

Contributed by Linda Broadhead
Third place, pH Miracle 2004 Recipe Contest
Transitional Category

MAKES 2–3 DOZEN

2 cups almonds, soaked
3 cups pecans, soaked
4 cups freeze-dried coconut flakes (Wilderness Family Naturals)
1 tsp. almond flavoring, non-alcohol (Frontier)
1 tsp. SlimSweet or equivalent sweetener
¾ cup flaxseeds, ground
¼ cup flaxseeds, ground
4 Tbs. water

In food processor, pulse-chop almonds and pecans until finely ground. Place in large mixing bowl with other ingredients except ¼ cup ground flaxseeds and water. Mix ¼ cup ground flaxseeds with water and let sit to moisten several minutes, before adding to mixing bowl. Mix thoroughly. Prepare dehydrator. Pour out mixture onto Teflex sheets; placing another Teflex sheet on top, use rolling pin to fatten about ¼-inch thick. Score with chopstick in shape of bars. Dehydrate at 100 degrees F for 9 hours. Transfer to mesh sheets, turning over bars. Dehydrate until fully dry, at least several more hours. Store in airtight container.

Molly's Crackers

Contributed by Linda Broadhead
Third place, pH Miracle 2004 Recipe Contest
Transitional Category

MAKES ABOUT 2 DOZEN

4 carrots
3 stalks celery
1 red pepper
2 cups pecans, soaked overnight
3 cups flaxseeds, ground
3 Tbs. sun-dried tomatoes, packed in oil
1 Tbs. RealSalt
Water, if necessary

In food processor, finely chop veggies and pecans. Add ground flaxseeds, sun-dried tomatoes, and salt. Process until well mixed. Prepare dehydrator. Place Teflex sheet on flat surface. Place ⅓ of the mixture in center of sheet. Cover with another Teflex sheet, using rolling pin to flatten mixture on sheet to ¼ inch. Score mixture with dull knife, into cracker-sized pieces. Dehydrate at 100 degrees F for 9 hours. Turn, and dehydrate additional 4 hours. Store in airtight container.

Morning Glory Crackers

Contributed by Eric Prouty
First place, pH Miracle 2004 Recipe Contest
Alkalizing Category

MAKES 2–3 DOZEN

4 cups dry sunflower seeds
1 cup dry flaxseeds

½ **bunch kale, spines removed**
½ **lb. carrots, peeled**
12 **bunches celery**
½ **head broccoli, including peeled stem**
¼ **head cabbage**
½ **onion**
2 **zucchini**
1¼ **cup pure water**
1 **Tbs. garlic**
1 **Tbs. RealSalt**
2 **Tbs. curry**
1 **Tbs. Bragg Liquid Aminos**

Soak sunflower seeds for 4 hours. Drain and puree in food processor. Set aside. Make flour with flaxseeds in blender or coffee grinder. Set aside. Chop kale in ½-inch pieces and place in large bowl. In food processor, pulse-chop carrots separately. Continue with remaining vegetables in batches, adding ¼ cup water, if needed. Place all into large bowl. Stir in seasonings and Braggs Liquid Aminos. Add balance of water to flaxseed flour and mix with vegetables completely. Add sunflower seeds and mix completely. Prepare dehydrator. Spread mixture smoothly onto Teflex sheets. Score into crackers. Dehydrate at 115 degrees F for 4 or 5 hours. Flip crackers and continue dehydrating at 105 degrees F until crisp (approximately 25 hours total).

Variations:
- For sweeter mild cracker reduce Bragg Liquid Aminos and salt. Replace curry with 1 Tbs. coriander and 1 Tbs. Tandori Blend (Spice Hunter).
- For garlic lovers, replace curry with extra 1 Tbs. garlic and 1 tsp. black pepper.

Peppermint Mana Delights

Contributed by Debra Jenkins
Second place, pH Miracle 2004 Recipe Contest
Alkalizing Category

MAKES 12

1 (5.4 oz.) Earth Essence Clay
5 Tbs. soy sprouts (¼ cup)
1 Tbs. SuperGreens powder
⅓ cup freeze-dried coconut flakes (Wilderness Family Naturals)
¼ tsp. peppermint flavoring, non-alcoholic (Frontier)

Mix together all ingredients. Form 1 tsp. of mixture into a small ball and roll in more coconut flakes to coat. Freeze for 30 minutes before serving. Store in freezer.

Raw Slim Sticks

Contributed by Debra Wanger Yaruss

MAKES 2–3 DOZEN

¼ cup raw organic sunflower seeds
¼ cup raw organic sesame seeds
¼ cup raw organic pumpkin seeds
½ cup raw organic almonds
1 tsp. RealSalt
3 Tbs. Italian seasoning (Spice Hunter)
7 sun-dried tomatoes
Juice of half a lemon or lime
6 raw dried Nori sheets, cut in half

Soak sunflower seeds, sesame seeds, pumpkin seeds, and almonds overnight to soften. Rinse seeds and nuts. Drain well. In food

processor, pulse-chop, then blend, sprouted seeds and almonds with RealSalt, Italian seasoning, sun-dried tomatoes, and lemon or lime until it is the consistency of thick paste. Cut Nori sheets in half and prepare flat surface to roll Slim Sticks. Spread 1 or 2 Tbs. of seed mixture into edge of Nori sheet as to roll sushi. Roll into tight little cigar shape. Brush with a bit of water to seal edges of sheet. Dehydrate on Teflex sheets at 112 degrees F for 2 to 3 days or until only slightly soft.

Variation:

- Add Mexican, curry, Jamaican jerk, or any other favorite seasoning combinations instead of Italian seasonings used in mixture.

Saladacco Veggie Crisps

SERVES 4–8

These curly veggie crisps are flavor-packed crunchies, made with the Saladacco, and then dehydrated. Use in the place of salad croutons, soup toppers, or to pop in your mouth for a true alkalarian snack, perfect for travel too. Experiment with different seasonings and marinades to make them different each time. If you don't have a Saladacco, a mandoline or a peeler will also work to get thin slices of the veggies.

2 yams (sweet potatoes work, or 4 carrots)
2 zucchini
1 large lemon, juiced
2 Tbs. olive oil
1 tsp. RealSalt (or to taste)
1 Tbs. Café Sol Seasoning (Spice Hunter), mixture of toas
  onion, mustard, and pure sea salt

Peel yam/sweet potatoes and cut into 2-inch pieces with pa horizontal ends. Process the yam pieces in the Saladacco o

curly position. Also process the zucchini the same way. However, you don't need to peel if they are organic. Place curlies in a shallow bowl and marinate for an hour or two in marinade of choice. Add lemon oil, salt, or spices of choice to marinade. You can even marinate them overnight in the fridge. When marinade is done, drain curlies and place on dehydrator sheets with net liners. Make sure not to overlap them. Dehydrate 6 to 12 hours until desired consistency (longer will give more of a chip crispness). Store in airtight containers.

Variations:
- Add ¼–½ cup sun-dried tomato bits to the marinade (I used packed in oil and process them into bits in the Cuisinart).
- Use fajita seasonings instead of Café Sol.
- Use mesquite seasonings instead of Café Sol.
- For a sweet version, instead of using the lemon juice and olive oil, marinate the curlies in the water of a Thai coconut and add two handfuls of Wilderness Family Farms freeze-dried coconut.
- You can also use other vegetables like carrots, beets, jicama, and squash.

Sandy's Almond Joy

Contributed by Sandy Kuntz
Honorable Mention, pH Miracle 2003 Recipe Contest

MAKES 12

1 cup almonds, soaked, chopped, dehydrated
1 tsp. RealSalt
1 cup liquid coconut oil
¾–1 cup dried coconut flakes (Wilderness Family Naturals preferred)
2–3 scoops soy sprouts powder (optional)

Soak almonds overnight in pure water and RealSalt to cover, refrigerate. Chop almonds. Place in dehydrator for 4 to 6 hours. Stir

together coconut oil, almonds, and dried coconut flakes, reserving half of dried coconut flakes for topping. Spread mixture in an 8 × 8-inch pan. Sprinkle remaining dried coconut flakes on top. Place in refrigerator for 45 minutes to 1 hour to chill (pan needs to be level for oil to distribute equally). Remove and cut into squares. If oil has chilled too much, set out at room temperature until bars can be easily cut.

Shelley's Variation: Add ½ tsp. vanilla extract. Try other flavorings such as banana or mint.

Savory Alkalarian Crackers

Contributed by Eric Prouty
First place, pH Miracle 2004 Recipe Contest
Alkalizing Category

MAKES 2–3 DOZEN

4 cups golden flaxseeds
1 Tbs. garlic
½ cup parsley
½ cup basil
1 tsp. cayenne powder
1 tsp. soaked caraway seeds
1 Tbs. RealSalt
5¼ cups warm water
1 Tbs. Bragg Liquid Aminos

In blender, on high, grind flaxseeds 1 cup at a time until most seeds are flour. Transfer to bowl. Add dry ingredients and mix. Add water and Bragg Liquid Aminos. Stir completely. Prepare dehydrator. Spread mixture ¼-inch thick onto Teflex sheets. Score into crackers. Dehydrate at 105 degree F for approximately 2 days.

Variations:
- Add ½ cup soaked sunflower seeds
- Add more soaked caraway seeds
- Add ½ cup diced onion and 1 tsp. Herbes de Provence

Sprouted Lentil Crackers

Contributed by Marlene Grauwels
First place, pH Miracle 2004 Recipe Contest
Alkalizing Category

MAKES 2–3 DOZEN

2 cups sunflower seeds, soaked 8–10 hours, sprouted 4 hours
2 cups green lentils, sprouted
½ cup golden flaxseeds, finely ground
4–6 carrots, finely grated
4 celery stalks, coarsely chopped
2–3 garlic cloves, chopped
2 green onions, chopped
4–6 Tbs. cilantro, chopped (parsley can be substituted)
2 tsps. Celtic Salt or RealSalt
1 Tbs. poultry seasoning
2 tsps. fresh oregano (or 1 tsp. dried)

In food processor, combine all ingredients. Pulse-chop, then blend thoroughly, in two separate batches. Prepare dehydrator. Place Cracker "dough" onto Teflex sheets spread very thin (about ¼-inch thick). Score with pizza cutter. Dehydrate for 8 to 12 hours. Store in airtight container.

Sweetarts and Sweetart Macaroons

SERVES 6–8

This is an alkalarian treat that is yummy, chewy, and energy packed. The sweet side of this great snack is full of healthy calcium, phosphorus, and magnesium, from the almonds, coconut, and coconut water. Ruby Red grapefruit with lycopene provides the tartness. It's great for travel and for those times when you just gotta have a munchy.

Note: *This recipe would be too sweet for someone suffering with a state of imbalance or yeast imbalances; however once healed and in balance, this recipe could be used occasionally for a treat.*

3 large ripe Ruby Red grapefruits, cut into 6 halves
Water from 1 young Thai coconut, crack and drain
1 heaping cup of freeze-dried shredded coconut (Wilderness Family Naturals)
2 cups almonds, soaked and plumped
Coconut meat from Thai coconut (optional—add this for more fresh coconut appeal)

Cut grapefruit in half and with a serrated-edged knife, slice around each section to separate it from the skin membrane. With a spoon, carefully scoop out all sections of grapefruit and place them in a bowl. (Save extra grapefruit juice to drink or use in a shake later.) Open the Thai coconut and drain the coconut water into a glass. There is a soft spot on the bottom of these coconuts where you can sink a knife or clean screwdriver and drain the water. Make sure the water is clear and sweet to the taste; it should not be fizzy, cloudy, or fermented. Strain out any wood pulp from the coconut water and pour over the grapefruit sections. Let the sections soak in the coconut water for a few minutes. Place freeze-dried coconut flakes in a bowl for dipping. Take soaked grapefruit sections, one at a time, and roll them into the coconut to heavily coat. Or push a soaked almond into the middle of the grapefruit section and then coat with the freeze-dried coconut for a nuttier crunch. Prepare dehydrator. Set grapefruit sections on a dehydrator tray lined with a screened (one with holes) sheet. Dehydrate overnight at 110 degrees F (or to desired crispness). Yummy chewy Sweetart treats!

Sweetart Macaroons

In a Cuisinart food processor, place drained soaked almonds, grapefruit sections (that have soaked in the coconut water), and freeze-dried coconuts. Process until you have a chunky wet mush (not too long). Spread out onto a Teflex-coated sheet about ½-inch thick, and dehydrate at 110 degrees F overnight. Check mixture after 12 hours; it should turn out pliable and chewy. If you desire a crisper macaroon, dehydrate longer. Break into large chunky pieces (about the size of a cookie) or score with a knife while drying to make more uniform shapes. Keep in Ziploc bags or Tupperware for storage (that's if there are any left after you pull them off the tray). Enjoy! Feel free to adjust ingredients to your liking each time you make this. You will probably have some grapefruit juice and coconut water leftover. Drink it later, use it in a shake, or freeze it into a Popsicle.

Variations:
• Instead of grapefruit sections, use *raw yams* that have been peeled and sliced very thin with a vegetable peeler (in long strips or chip-style) or sliced into thin spirals with the Saladacco. Soak the thinly sliced yams in the coconut water for a few minutes and then roll them in the freeze-dried coconut to coat them. Dehydrate overnight or to desired crispness. These make wonderful pop-in-the-mouth snacks or really great sweet croutons for your next salad. If desired, soak any kind of nuts (almonds, pecans, sunflower seeds, walnuts, etc.) in the coconut water, roll them in the freeze-dried coconut, and re-dehydrate them. Great salad or soup toppers or snacks. Enjoy!

Resources

The pH Miracle
The pH Miracle Living Centers
16390 Dia Del Sol
Valley Center, CA 92082
760-751-8321
Fax: 760-751-8324
www.phmiracleliving.com
   Call for referrals for live blood analysis and the Mycotoxic/
Oxidative Stress Test (MOST), or health retreats or consultations,
and information not covered in this section about products mentioned in this book. Or check out these websites:
   www.thephmiraclecenter.com or www.phmiracleliving.com
   For general information and information about Needak rebounders, pH paper, and more, including workshops on preparing alkalizing meals through Shelley Young's Academy of Culinary Arts.
   www.thephmiracle.us or www.phmiracleliving.com
   For general information, articles, and testimonials, as well as
more information on the Plasma Activated Electro-Magnetic Mi-
croIonization Water Machine.
   www.thephmiracleliving.com and www.phmiracleliving.com
   For pH Miracle Living Nutritionals (supplements), the Regenesis
Water Machine, videos on the New Biology and the pH Miracle lifestyle and diet, and information about The pH Miracle Living Foundation, which is dedicated to children with serious health challenges,

including obesity, and helping them and their parents with alternative health education.

www.phmiracleliving.com

For organically grown California avocados, picked fresh off the tree and shipped to you next day.

Organizations

Physicians Committee for Responsible Medicine
5100 Wisconsin Avenue, NW
Suite 404
Washington, DC 20016
202-686-2210
www.perm.org

Promotes preventative medicine, encourages higher standards for ethics and effectiveness in research, and advocates broader access to medical services.

Citizens for Health
P.O. Box 2260
Boulder, CO 80306
800-357-2211
www.citizens.org

Empowers consumers to make informed health choices in the areas of dietary supplements, complementary and alternative medicine, food and water safety.

Food and Water Journal and Wild Matters
389 Route 215
Walden, VT 05873
800-EAT-SAFE
www.foodandwater.org

Leads tenacious and effective public campaigns against toxic food and water technologies, including food irradiation, pesticides, and genetically modified organisms (GMOs), while stimulating efforts to build safe, sustainable alternatives.

International Vegetarian Union
P.O. Box 9710
Washington, DC 20016
202-362-VEGY
www.ivu.org
   Promotes vegetarianism throughout the world by supporting and connecting national and regional groups, and holding International Vegetarian Congress.

North American Vegetarian Society (NAVS)
P.O. Box 72
Dolgeville, NY 13329
518-568-7970
www.navs-online.org
   Dedicated to promoting the vegetarian way of life by sponsoring regional and national conferences and campaigns, distributing educational materials, and publishing *Vegetarian Voice*.

Food

Garden of Life
800-622-8986
www.gardenoflifeusa.com
   For extra-virgin coconut oil.

Manitoba Harvest
Hemp Foods and Oils
Winnipeg, Manitoba, Canada
R3H OK2
800-665-HEMP
www.manitobaharvest.com
   For cold-pressed hemp and pumpkin oils.

New Frontier
www.frontiercoop.com
   For flavorings bottled in oil (without alcohol).

Workstead Industries
P.O. Box 1083
Greenfield, MA 01302
413-772-6816
  For Pomona's Universal Pectin.

The Cape Herb and Spice Company
Distributed by Profile Products
P.O. Box 140
Maple Valley, WA 98038
425-432-4300
www.elements-of-spice.com
  For Heat Wave seasoning.

Lite House Spice Company
www.litehousefoods.com

Spice House
www.thespicehouse.com
  For dehydrated tomato powder and veggie granules.

Mauk Family Farms
www.Maukfamilyfarms.com
  For raw wheat-free crusts.

Redmond Minerals, Inc.
800-367-7258
www.realsalt.com
  For RealSalt.

Life Sprouts
P.O. Box 150
Hiram, UT 94321
435-245-3891
  For a wonderful, easy-to-get-started program on sprouting, kits
in different sizes, instructions on how to sprout, information on nutritional aspects of different seeds, single seeds, and seed mixes.

Diamond Organics
P.O. Box 2159
Freedom, CA 95019
888-674-2642
Fax orders: 888-888-6777
e-mail: organics@diamondorganics.com
　There are many organic food distributors, many of which are based in California due to the year-round growing climate; this is one I like.

Pacific Foods
19480 SW 97th Avenue
Tualatin, OR 97062
503-692-9666
www.pacificfoods.com
　For yeast-free vegetable broth.

Flora, Inc.
Lyden, WA 98264
800-446-2110
www.udoerasmus.com
www.florainc.com
　For Udo's Choice.

Barlean's Organic Oils
4936 Lake Terrell Road
Ferndale, WA 98248
800-445-FLAX
　Look for this cold-pressed oil in the refrigerator case of your local natural foods store.

Arrowhead Mills
Vancouver, BC V5L 1P5
800-661-3529
www.omeganutrition.com
　For Essential Balance/Omega Nutrition Oil.

Blue Moon Acres
2237 Durham Road (RTE. 413)
Buckingham, PA 18912
215-794-3093
    For locally grown organic specialty salad greens formerly available only to the finest chefs but now available to the general public.

Image Foods, Inc.
350 Cambridge Avenue, Suite 350
Palo Alto, CA 94306
www.imagefoods.com

Pomi
www.foodservicedirect.com
    For strained tomatoes with no preservatives, additives, or vinegar.

White Wave
www.whitewave.com
    For baked seasoned tofu and other tofu products.

Wisdom Herbs
Mesa, AZ 85202
800-899-9908
www.wisdomherbs.com
www.steviaplus.com
    For SweetLeaf Plus stevia with fiber.

Boca Burgers
www.bocaburger.com

Spice Hunter
www.spicehunter.com

Equipment

Cutting Edge Catalogue
P.O. Box 5034
Southampton, NY 11969
800-497-9516
516-287-3813
Fax: 516-287-3112
e-mail: cutcat@I-2000.com
www.cutcat.com
  For pH meters, water systems, books, and more.

Nova
www.novacompanies.com
  For infrared sauna.

Vita-Mix
8615 Usher Road
Cleveland, OH 44138-2199
800-848-2649
  For the blender with the plunger.

Green Power
888-254-7336
562-940-4240
www.greenpower.com
  For Green Star Green Life Juicer.

Crystal Clear
Westbrook Farms, Route 209
Westbrookville, NY 12785
800-433-9553
www.johnellis.com
  For the Living Water Machine.

Supplements

pH Miracle
16390 Dia Del Sol
Valley Center, CA 92082
760-751-8321
Fax: 760-751-8324
www.phmiracleliving.com
www.phmiraclenutrition.com

Green Kamut Corporation
1965 Freeman
Long Beach, CA 90804

InnerLight, Inc.
867 East 2260 South
Provo, UT 84606
www.innerlightinc.com

Nordic Naturals
54 Hangar Way
Watsonville, CA 95076
800-662-2544
www.nordicnaturals.com

Solaray Nutraceutical Corporation
1400 Kearns Boulevard, Second Floor
Park City, UT 84060
800-669-8877
www.nutraceutical.com

Source Natural, Inc.
19 Janis Way
Scotts Valley, CA 95066
800-815-2333
www.sourcenaturals.com

Think Thin

Laughter Yoga
www.laughteryoga.org

Books

The Blood and Its Third Anatomical Element by Antoine Bechamp
Clinical Physiology of Acid-Base and Electrolyte Disorders by Burton David Rose, M.D., and Theodore W. Post, M.D.
The Complete Book of Massage by Claire Maxwell Hudson
Fat Wars by Brad J. King
Fats That Heal and Fats That Kill by Udo Erasmus
Flax the Super Food by Barb Bloomfield, Judy Brown, and Siegfried Gursche
The Food Revolution by John Robbins
The Healing Miracles of Coconut Oil by Bruce Fife, N.D.
The Miracle of Magnesium by Carolyn Dean, M.D., N.D.
Molecules of Emotion by Candace B. Pert, Ph.D.
Muscles in Minutes by Mike Mentzer
A New Look at Coconut Oil by Mary G. Enig, Ph.D., FACN
The Oil-Protein Diet by Johanna Budwig, M.D.
The Omega Diet by Artemis P. Simopoulos, M.D., and Jo Robinson
Patient Heal Thyself by Jordon Rubin
Slow Burn by Stu Mittleman
Soy Smart Health by Neil Solomon, M.D., Ph.D.
Static Contraction by Peter Sisco and John Little
Taking Charge of Your Weight and Well-Being by Joyce D. Nash, Ph.D., and Linda H. Ormiston, Ph.D.
The Touch That Heals by William N. Brown, Ph.D., N.D., D.Sc.
The Trans Fat Solution by Kim Severson
Understanding Acid-Base by Benjamin Abelow, M.D.
Urban Rebounding by J. B. Berns
Water and Salt, The Essence of Life by Barbara Nendel, M.D.

Appendix

DAILY JOURNAL

Date:
Hours slept:
Overall energy levels:
Overall mood:
Daily health markers (optional):

Exercise:
Duration:

Alkaline Water: _____ liters
    How many liters were green drink (with green powder and
      pH drops)?
    How many liters had soy spouts? _____

Supplements:
Omega-3s and omega-6s: Dose:
L-carnitine: Dose:
Garcinia cambogia or HCA/chromium/tyrosine: Dose:
Clay: Dose:
Other: Dose:

Food:
Time: Food:

Emotions:
Notable feelings. Include any connection to what you
ate/drank/took:

References

Agatston, A. *The South Beach Diet: The Delicious, Doctor-Designed, Foolproof Plan for Fast and Healthy Weight Loss.* New York: Rodale, distributed by St. Martin's Press, 2003.

Ahluwalia, P., and Malik, V. B. Effects of monosodium glutamate (MSG) on serum lipids, blood glucose and cholesterol in adult male mice. *Toxicology Letters*, February 1989; 45(2–3): 195–98.

Allison, D., et al. Annual deaths attributable to obesity in the United States. *Journal of the American Medical Association*, 1999; 16: 1530–38.

CLA could help control weight, fat, diabetes, and muscle loss. *American Chemical Society National Meeting News*, August 20, 2000.

Microbial pollutants in our nation's water. *American Society for Microbiology*, Washington, DC, 1999.

Anderson, R. A., Effects of chromium on body composition and weight loss. *Nutrition Reviews*, 1998; 56(9): 266–70.

Andrews, J. F. Exercise for slimming. *Proceedings of the Nutrition Society*, August 1991; 50 (2): 459–71.

Atkins, R. *Dr. Atkins' New Diet Revolution.* New York: M. Evans & Co., 1999.

Badmaev, V., Majeed, M., and Conte, A. A. Garcinia cambogia for weight loss. *Journal of the American Medical Association*, 1999; 282: 233–34.

Banderet, L. E., and Lieberman, H. R. Treatment with tyrosine, a neurotransmitter precursor, reduces environmental stress in humans. *Brain Research Bulletin*, 1989; 22: 759–62.

Barilla, J. *Olive Oil Miracle: How the Mediterranean Marvel Helps Protect Against Arthritis, Heart Disease, and Breast Cancer.* New Canaan, CT: Keats Publishing, 1996.

Bar-Or, O., et al. Physical activity, genetic, and nutritional considerations in childhood weight management. *Medicine and Science in Sports and Exercise*, 1998; 30 (1): 2–10.

Batmanghelidj, F. *Your Body's Many Cries for Water.* Falls Church, VA: Global Health Solutions, 1998.

Baumgartner, R. N., et al. Association of fat and muscle masses with bone mineral in elderly men and women. *American Journal of Clinical Nutrition,* 1996; 63: 365.

Bellize, M. C., and Dietz, W. H. Workshop on childhood obesity: Summary of the discussion. *American Journal of Clinical Nutrition,* 1999 supplement; 70: 173S–175S.

Berns, J. B., with Flaum, J. *Urban Rebounding: An Exercise for the New Millennium.* New York: KE Publishing, 1999.

Better Business Bureau. *Tips for consumers: Safe drinking water.* The Council of Better Business Bureau, 4200 Wilson Blvd., Suite 800, Arlington, VA 22203-1838; 703-276-0100; www.bbb.org.

Blankson, H., et al. Conjugated linoleic acid reduces body fat mass in overweight and obese humans. *Journal of Nutrition,* 2000; 130: 2943–48.

Blaylock, R. L. *Excitotoxins: The Taste That Kills.* Sante Fe, NM: Health Press, 1997.

Bloomfield, B., Brown, J., and Gursche, S. *Flax: The Super Food!* Summertown, TN: Book Publishing Company, 2000.

Bouchard, C., et al. Inheritance of the amount and distribution of human body fat. *International Journal of Obesity,* 1988; 12: 205.

Brody, J. E. For life gains, just add water. *New York Times,* July 11, 2000.

Brooks, L. *Rebounding to Better Health: A Practical Guide to the Ultimate Exercise.* O'Neill, NE: KE Publishing, 1995, p. 15.

Bunyan, J. Murrell, E. A., and Shah, P. P. The induction of obesity in rodents by means of monosodium glutamate. *British Journal of Nutrition,* 1976; 35(1): 25–39.

Brown, L. Obesity epidemic threatens health in exercise-deprived countries. *Worldwatch Institute,* December 19, 2000.

Bruinsma, K., and Taren, D. L. Chocolate: Food or drug? *American Dietetic Association,* 1999; 10: 1249–56.

Brynr, R. W., et al. Effects of resistance vs. aerobic training combines with an 800 calorie liquid diet on lean body mass and resting metabolic rate. *Journal of the American College of Nutrition,* 1999; 18(2): 115–21.

Budwig, J. *The Oil-Protein Diet Cookbook.* Vancouver, Canada: Apple Publishing, 1994.

Bullers, A. Bottled water: Better than the tap? *FDA Consumer,* July–August 2002.

Burke, E. R. *Optimal Muscle Recovery.* New York: Avery Publishing Group, 1999.

Cameron, D. P., Cutbush, L., and Opat, F. Effects of monosodium glutamate-induced obesity in mice on carbohydrate metabolism in insulin secretion. *Clinical and Experimental Pharmacology and Physiology,* January–February 1978; 5(1): 41–51.

Caprio, S., et al. Metabolic impact of obesity in childhood. *Endocrinology Metabolism Clinics of North America,* 1999; 28(4): 731–47.

Carlson, L. A., et al. Studies on blood lipids during exercise. *Journal of Laboratory and Clinical Medicine,* 1963; 61: 724–29.

Carter, A. E. *The New Miracles of Rebound Exercise: A Revolutionary Way to Better Health and Fitness.* Fountain Hills, AZ: A.L.M. Publishers, 1988, p. 38.

Castleman, M. *The Healing Herbs.* New York: Bantam, 1995.

Cheema-Dhadli, S., Harlperin, M. L., and Leznoff, C. C. Inhibition of enzymes which interact with citrate by (-)hydroxycitrate and 1,2,3, -tricarboxybenzene. *European Journal of Biochemistry,* 1973; 38: 98–102.

Cherniske, S. *Caffeine Blues.* New York: Warner Books, 1998.

Chilibeck, P. D., et al. Higher mitochondrial fatty acid oxidation following intermittent versus continuous endurance exercise training. *Canadian Journal of Physiology and Pharmacology,* September 1998; 76(9): 891–94.

Clouet, P., et al. Effect of short and long term treatments by a low level dietary L-carnitine on parameters related to fatty acid oxidation in winstar rat. *Biochemica et Biophysica ACTA,* 1996; 1299(2): pp 191–97.

Colgan, M. *Antioxidants: The Real Story.* Vancouver, BC: Apple Publishing, 1998.

Colgan, M., and Colgan, L. *The Flavonoid Revolution.* Vancouver, BC: Apple Publishing, 1997.

Conacher, D. *Troubled Waters on Tap: Organic Chemicals in Public Drinking Water Systems and the Failure of Regulation.* Washington, DC: Center for Study of Responsive Law, 1988.

Conley, E. *America Exhausted.* Flint, MI: Valley Press, 1998.

Coyne, L. L. *Fat Won't Make You Fat.* Alberta: Fish Creek Publishing, 1998.

Crawford, P., et al. How can Californians be overweight and hungry? *California Agriculture,* January–March, 2004; 58(1).

Cutting, T. M., et al. Like mother, like daughter, familial patterns of overweight are mediated by mothers' dietary disinhibition. *American Journal of Clinical Nutrition,* 1999; 69(4): 608–13.

D'Adama, P. J. *Eat Right for Your Type.* New York: Putman, 1996.

Danbrot, M. *The New Cabbage Soup Diet.* New York: St. Martin's Paperbacks, 2004.

Daoust, G., and Daoust, J. *40–30–30 Fat Burning Nutrition: The Dietary Hormonal Connection to Permanent Weight Loss and Better Health.* Del Mar, CA: Wharton Publishing, 1996.

Dean, C. *The Miracle of Magnesium.* London: Simon & Schuster, 2003.

Diamond, H., and Diamond, M. *Fit for Life.* New York: Warner Books, 1985.

Drinker, C. K., and Yoffey, J. M. *Lymphatics, Lymph, and Lymphoid Tissue.* Cambridge, MA: Harvard University Press, 1941, pp. 17–19.

Dufty, W. *Sugar Blues.* New York: Warner Books, 1975.

Eades, M. R., and Eades, M. D. *Protein Power.* New York: Bantam Books, 1999.

Eaton, S. B. Humans, lipids and evolution. *Lipids,* 1992; 27(10): 814–20.

Eaton, S. B., et al. An evolutionary perspective enhances understanding of human nutritional requirements. *Journal of Nutrition,* June 1996; 126: 1732–40.

Elkins, R. *Stevia: Nature's Sweetener.* Pleasant Grove, UT: Woodland Publishing, 1997.

Enig, M. G. *Know Your Fats: The Complete Primer for Understanding the Nutrition of Fats, Oils, and Cholesterol.* Colorado Springs, CO: Healthwise Publications, 2000.

Epstein, S. S., and Zavon, M. Is there a threshold for cancer? In *International Water Quality Symposium: Water—Its Effects of Life Quality,* ed. D. Manners. Washington, DC: Water Quality Research Council, 1974, 54–62.

Ezin, C., with Caron, K. *Your Fat Can Make You Thin.* New York: Contemporary Books, 2000.

Fallon, S., and Enig, M. Tragedy and hype, the third international soy symposium. *Nexus Magazine,* April–May 2000; 7(3).

Fife, B. *Eat Fat Look Thin: A Safe and Natural Way to Lose Weight Permanently.* Colorado Springs, CO: Healthwise Publications, 2002.

Fife, B. *The Healing Miracles of Coconut Oil.* Colorado Springs, CO: Healthwise Publications, 2003.

Fox, M. *Healthy Water for a Longer Life.* Portsmouth, NH: Healthy Water Research, 1990, pp. 12–14.

Fraci, S. *The Power of SuperFoods: 30 Days That Will Change Your Life.* Toronto: Prentice Hall, Canada, 1997.

Friedman, J. M. Obesity in the new milleninium. *Nature,* 2000; 404(6778): 632–34.

Galbo, H. Endocrinology and metabolism in exercise. *International Journal of Sports Medicine,* 1981; 2: 125.

Gelenberg, A. J., Gibson, C. J., and Wojcik, J. D. Neurotransmitter precursors for the treatment of depression. *Psychopharmacology Bulletin*, 1982; 18: 7–18.

Germano, C. *Advantra Z: The Natural Way to Lose Weight Safely.* New York: Kensington, 1998.

Ghorbam, M., et al. Hypertrophy of brown adipocytes in brown and white adipose tissues and reversal of diet induced obesity in rats treated with a beta-3 adrenoceptor agonist. *Biochemistry Pharmacology*, 1997; 54: 121–31.

Golan, M. I., et al. Parents as the exclusive agents of change in the treatment of childhood obesity. *American Journal of Clinical Nutrition*, 1998; 67(6): 1130–35.

Golay, A., et al. Weight-loss with low or high carbohydrate diet? *International Journal of Obesity and Related Metabolic Disorders*, 1996; 20(12): 1067–72.

Goodman, E. We should strive to drive less to get out of fat city. *Contra Costa Times*, February 10, 2004.

Gorman, J. Beware the funky chicken. Special Report, *Men's Health*, April 4, 2004; 104–10.

Graci, S. *The Food Connection.* Toronto: Macmillan Canada, 2001.

Grant, K. E., et al. Chromium and exercise training: Effect on obese women. *Medicine and Science in Sports and Exercise*, 1997; 29(8): 992–98.

Grant, W. B. Low fat, high-sugar diet and lipoprotein profiles. *American Journal of Clinical Nutrition*, 1999; 70(6): 1111–12.

Greenwood, M. R. C., Cleary, M. P., Gruen, R., et al. Effect of (-)-hydroxycitrate on development of obesity in the Zucker obese rat. *American Journal of Physiology*, 1981; 240: E72–78.

Guezennec, C. Y. Role of lipids on endurance capacity in man. *International Journal of Sports Medicine*, 1992; 13(suppl. 1): S114–S118.

Gura, T. Uncoupling proteins provide new clue to obesity's causes. *Science*, May 29, 1998; 280: 1369–70.

Gutman, J. *Glutathione: Its Role in Cancer & Anticancer Therapy.* Canada: Health Books, 2002.

Hamaoka, K., and Kusunoki, T. Morphological and cell proliferative study on the growth of visceral organs in monosodium L-glutamate-treated obese mice. *Journal of Nutritional Science and Vitaminology* (Tokyo). August 1986; 32(4): 395–411.

Harper, M. E. Obesity research continues to spring leaks. *Clinical and Investitative Medicine*, August 20, 1998; 239–244.

Harris, W. S., et al. Influence of n-3 fatty acid supplementation on the endogenous activities of plasma lipae. *American Journal of Clinical Nutrition*, 1997; 66(2): pp 254–60.

Heleniak, E., and Aston, B. Prostaglandins, brown fat and weight loss. *Medical Hypotheses*, 1989; 28: 13–33.

Heller, R., and Heller, R. *The Carbohydrate Addict's Program for Success.* New York: Penguin Publishing, 1993.

Hendel, B., and Ferreira, P. *Water & Salt, The Essence of Life.* Natural Resources, 2003.

Heymsfield, S. B., Allison, D. B., Vasselli, J. R., et al. Garcinia cambogia (hydroxycitric acid) as a potential antiobesity agent. *Journal of the American Medical Association*, 1998; 280: 1596–1600.

Hirata, A. E., Andrade, I. S., Vaskevicius, P., and Dolnikoff, M.S. Monosodium glutamate (MSG)-obese rats develop glucose intolerance and insulin resistance to peripheral glucose uptake. *Brazilian Journal of Medical and Biological Research*, May 1997; 30(5): 671–74.

Hirose, Y., Ishihara, K., Terashi, K., Kazumi, T., Utsumi, M., Morita, S., and Baba, S. Hypothalamic obesity induced by monosodium glutamate (MSG) in rats: Changes in the endocrine pancreas in the course of and after induction obesity. *Nippon Naibunpi Gakkai Zasshi*, February 20, 1983; 59(2): 196–207.

Horrocks, L. S., and Leo, Y. K. Health benefits of docosahexaenoic acid (DHA). *Pharmacological Research*, 1999; 40(3): 211–24.

Kaats, G. R. Effects of multiple herbal formulation on body composition, blood chemistry, vital signs and self-reported energy levels and appetitie control. *International Journal of Obesity*, 1994.

Kaats, G. R., et al. A randomized double-masked, placebo-controlled study of the effects of chromium picolinate supplementation on body composition: A replication and extension of a previous study. *Current Therapeutic Research*, 1998; 59: 379–88.

Kaats, G. R., Blum, K., Fisher, J. A., and Adelman, J. A. Effects of chromium picolinate supplementation on body composition: A randomized, double-masked, placebo-controlled study. *Current Therapeutic Research*, October 1996; 57(10): 747.

Kataria, M. *Laugh for No Reason.* Madhuri International, Andheri, Mumbai, 2002; www.laughteryoga.org.

Key, T., el al. Prevalence of obesity is low in people who do not eat meat. *British Medical Journal*; 1996; 313: 816–17.

Kishi, Y., et al. Alpha-lipoic acid: Effect on glucose uptake, sorbitol pathway, and energy metabolism in experimental diabetic ceuropathy. *Diabetes*, 1999; 48(10): 2045–51.

Klein, S. The war against obesity: Attacking a new front. *American Journal of Clinical Nutrition*, June 1999; 69(6): 1061–63.

Knopper, M. Water is becoming a dangerous drug. *E* magazine, December, 2002.

Knudsen, C. Super soy: Health benefits of soy protein. *Energy Times*, February 1996; 12.

Krinsky, N. I., et al. Antioxidant vitamins and beta-carotene in disease prevention. *American Journal of Clinical Nutrition*, 1995; 6(S): 1229S–1540S.

Kronberger, H., and Lattacher, S. *On the Track of Water's Secret.* Hamberg, Germany: *Wiener Verlag,* 1995.

Kushner, R., and Kushner, N. *Dr. Kushner's Personality Type Diet.* New York: St. Martin's Press, 2003.

Kwiterovich, P. O., Jr. The effect of dietary fat, antioxidants, and pro-oxidants on blood, lipids, lipoproteins, and atherosclerosis. *Journal of the American Dietetic Association*, 1997 (7 Suppl.): S31–41.

Langcuster, J., and Hairston, J. *Cryptosporidium: A Cause of Mounting Concern Among Water Authorities.* Alabama A & M and Auburn Universities.

Lawrence, J., et al. High fat, low carbs, what's the harm. *CBS Healthwatch, Medscape,* December 1999.

Lee, D. *Essential Fatty Acids: The "Good" Fats.* Pleasant Grove, UT: Woodland Publishing, 1997.

Lemonick, M. Why we grew so big. Special Issue. *TIME,* June 7, 2004; 163(23):, 57–69.

Lieberman, H. R., Corkin, S., Spring, B. J., Wurtman, R. J., and Growden, J. H. The effects of dietary neurotransmitter precursors on human behavior. *American Journal of Clinical Nutrition,* 1985; 42: 366–70.

Lorden, J. F., and Caudle, A. Behavioral and endocrinological effects of single injections of monosodium glutamate in the mouse. *Neurobehavioral Toxicology and Teratology,* September–October 1986; 8(5): 509–19.

Lorden, J. F., and Sims, J. S. Monosodium L-glutamate lesions reduce susceptibility to hypoglycemic feeding and convulsions. *Behavioral Brain Research,* May 1987; 24(2): 139–46.

Lowenstein J. M. Effect of (-)-hydroxycitrate on fatty acid synthesis by rat liver *in vivo. Journal of Biological Chemistry,* 1971; 246: 629–32.

Lowenstein, J. M. Experiments with (-)hydroxycitrate. In *Essays in Cell Metabolism,* ed. W. Burtley, H. L. Kornberg, and J. R. Quayle. New York: Wiley Interscience, 1970, pp. 153–66.

Lurz, R., and Fischer, R. *Aerztezeitschrift fur Naturheilverfahren,* 1998; 39: 12.

Markert, D. *The Turbo-Protein Diet.* Houston: BioMed International, 1999.

Marks, W. E. *The Holy Order of Water: Healing Earth's Waters and Ourselves.* Great Barrington, MA: Bell Ponds Books, 2001, pp. 173–80, 143–44, and 202–4.

McCartney, N. A., et al. Usefullness of weightlifting training in improving strength and maximal power output in coronary artery disease. *American Journal of Cardiology,* 1991; 67: 939.

McCarty, M. F. Vegan proteins may reduce risk of cancer, obesity, and cardiovascular disease by promoting increased glucagon activity. *Medical Hypotheses,* 1999; 53(6): 459–85.

McCrory, M. A., et al. Overeating in America: Association between restaurant food consumption and body fatness in healthy adult men and women ages 19 to 80. *Obesity Research,* 1999; 7(6): 564–71.

McGarry, J., and Foster, D. Regulation of hepatic fatty acid production and ketone body production. *Annual Review of Biochemistry,* 1980; 49: 395–420.

McGee, C. T. *Heart Frauds: Uncovering the Biggest Health Scam in History.* Colorado Springs, CO: Healthwise Publications, 2001.

McGraw, P. *The Ultimate Weight Solution: The 7 Keys to Weight Loss Freedom.* New York: The Free Press, 2003.

Mercola, J. *The NO-Grain Diet: Conquer Carbohydrate Addiction and Stay Slim for Life.* New York: Penguin Group (USA), 2003.

Messina, M. J., et al. Second International Symposium on the Role of Soy in Preventing and Treating Chronic Diseases, Brussels, September 19, 1996; 36.

Meyer, J. S., Welch, K. M. A., Deshmuckh, V. D., et al. Neurotransmitter precursor amino acids in the treatment of multi-infarct dementia and Alzheimer's disease. *Journal of the American Geriatric Society,* 1977; 7: 289–98.

Meyerowitz, S. *Wheat Grass, Nature's Finest Medicine.* Great Barrington, MA: The Sprout House, 1999.

Meyerowitz, S. *Water: The Ultimate Cure.* Tennessee Book Publishing Company, 2001, p. 46.

Miller, J. B., et al. *The New Glucose Revolution: The Authoritative Guide to the Glycemic Index—The Dietary Solution for Lifelong Health.* New York: Marlowe & Company, 2003.

Miller, P. M. *The Hilton Head Over-35 Diet.* New York: Warner Books, 1989.

Miller, P. M. *The New Hilton Head Metabolism Diet.* New York: Warner Books, 1996.

Mindel, E. *Earl Mindell's Soy Miracle.* New York: Simon & Schuster, 1995.

Mirkin, G., and Fox, B. *20/30 Fat & Fiber Diet Plan: The Weight-Reducing, Health-Promoting Nutrition System for Life.* New York: HarperCollins, 1998.

Mori, T. A., et al. Dietary fish as a major component of a weight-loss diet: Effect on serum lipids, glucose and insulin metabolism in overweight hypertensive subjects. *American Journal of Clinical Nutrition,* 1999; 70(5): 818–25.

Morter, M. T., M.S., D.C. *Correlative Urinalysis.* Rogers, AR: Best Research, 1988.

Nash, J. D., and Ormiston, L. H. *Taking Charge of Your Weight and Well-Being.* Palo Alto, CA: Bull Publishing, 1978.

National Resources Defense Council. *Bottled Water: Pure Drink or Pure Hype.* New York: NRDC, February 1999.

Nelson, G. J., Schmidt, P. C., and Kelley, D.S. Low-fat diets do not lower plasma cholesterol levels in healthy men compared to high-fat diets with similar fatty acid composition at constant calorie intake. *Lipids,* 1996; 31(Suppl.): S271–S274.

Newman, C. Why are we so fat? *National Geographic,* August 2004; 46–61.

Nikoletseas, M. M. Obesity in exercising, hypophagic rats treated with monosodium glutamate. *Physiology and Behavior,* December 1977; 19(6): 767–73.

Nishimura, O. Brain development in the symptomatic obesity model mouse with brain dysfunction. II. Dendritic development of neurons in the cerebral cortex. *No To Hattatsu.* November 1987; 19(6): 460–9.

Null, G. *Ultimate Lifetime Diet: A Revolutionary All-Natural Program for Losing Weight and Building a Healthy Body.* New York: Broadway Books, 2000.

Ochi, M., Fukuhara, K., Sawada, T., Hattori, T., and Kusunoki, T. Development of the epididymal adipose tissue in monosodium glutamate-induced obese mice. *Journal of Nutrition and Science Vitaminology* (Tokyo), June 1988; 34(3): 317–26.

Olney, J. W. Brain lesions, obesity, and other disturbances in mice treated with monosodium glutamate. *Science,* May 9, 1969; 164(880): 719–21. No abstract available.

Ornish, D. *Eat More, Weigh Less: Dr. Dean Ornish's Program for Losing Weight Safely While Eating Abundantly.* New York: HarperCollins Publishers, 2001.

Owen, K., et al. *Swine Day.* University of Nebraska, 1994; 161.

Owen, K., et.al. *Swine Day Rep. I.* University of Nebraska, 1996.

Packer, L., and Colman, C. *The Antioxidant Miracle.* New York: John Wiley & Sons, 1998.

Partiza, M. W., Park, Y., and Cook, M. E. Mechanism of action of conjugated linoleic acid: Evidence and speculation. *Proceedings of the Society for Experimental Biology and Medicine*, 2000; 233: 8–13.

Passwater, R. *Fish Oil Update: Latest Research on Marine Lipids and Their Newly Discovered Health Roles*. New Canaan, CT: Keats Publishing, 1987.

Patterson, C. R. *Essentials of Biochemistry*. London: Pittman Books, 1983, p. 38.

Paulson, D. J., et al. Carnitine deficiency-induced cardiomyopathy. *Molecular and Cellular Biochemistry*, 1998; 180: 33–41.

Perls, T. T., and Hutter Silver, M., with Lauerman, J. F. *Living to 100: Lessons in Living to Your Maximum Potential at Any Age*. New York: Basic Books, 1999, p. 168.

Perrone, T. *Hollywood's Healthiest Diets: 10 Fat-Fighting Plans*. New York: Regan Books, HarperCollins Publishers, 1999.

Pert, C.B., *Molecules of Emotions, Why You Feel the Way You Feel*. London: Simon & Schuster UK, 1998.

Physicians Committee for Responsible Health. Atkins dieters report serious health problems. *Good Medicine*, Winter 2004; XIII(1): 6–7.

Physicians Committee for Responsible Health. Is beef safe? *Good Medicine*, Winter 2004; XIII(1): 2.

Physicians Committee for Social Responsibility. Drinking water and disease: What health care providers should know. Washington, DC, 2000; www.psr.org.

Pizzi, W. J., and Barnhart, J. E. Effects of monosodium glutamate on somatic development, obesity and activity in the mouse. *Pharmacology, Biochemistry and Behavior*, November 1976; 5(5): 551–57.

Pratt, S., and Matthews, K. *SuperFoods, Fourteen Foods That Will Change Your Life*. New York: Willow Morrow, an Imprint of HarperCollins Publishers, 2004.

Pressman, A. H. *Glutathione, The Ultimate Antioxidant*. New York: St. Martin's Press, 1998.

Rebouche, C. J., and Paulson, D. J. Carnitine metabolism and function in humans. *Annual Review of Nutrition*, 1986; 6: 41–66.

Remke, H., Wilsdorf, A., and Muller, F. Development of hypothalamic obesity in growing rats. *Experimental Pathology*, 1988; 33(4): 223–32.

Reyes, B., et al. Effects of L-carnitine on erythrocyte acyl-CoZ, free CoA, and glycerophospholipid acyltransferase in uremia. *American Journal of Clinical Nutrition*, 1998; 67(3): 386–90.

Richard, L. *The Secret to Low Carb Success! How to Get the Most Out of Your Low Carbohydrate Diet*. New York: Kensington Publishing, 2001.

Robbins, J. *The Food Revolution, How Your Diet Can Help Save Your Life and Our World.* Boston: Conari Press, 2001.

Robert, M. and Martin, M. D. *The Gravity Guiding System.* San Marino, CA: Essential Publishing, 1975, pp. 1–14.

Robinzon, B., Snapir, N., and Perek, M. The relation between monosodium glutamate-inducing brain damage, and body weight, food intake, semen production and endocrine criteria in the fowl. *Poultry Science,* January 1975; 54(1): 234–41.

Romanowski, W., and Grabiec, S. The role of serotonin in the mechanism of central fatigue. *ACTA Physiologica Polonica,* 1974; 25: 127–34.

Ross, J. *The Diet Cure: The 8-Step Program to Rebalance Your Body Chemistry and End Food Cravings, Weight Problems, and Mood Swings—Now.* New York: Penguin Books, 1999.

Rubin, J. *The Maker's Diet: The 40-Day Health Experience That Will Change Your Life Forever.* Lake Mary, FL: Siloam Press, 2004.

Ryrie, C. *The Healing Energies of Water.* Boston: Journey Editions, an imprint of Periplus Editions (HK) Ltd., 1999, p. 56.

Salas, S. J. Influence of adiposity on the thermic effect of food and exercise in lean and obese adolescents. *International Journal of Obesity and Metabolic Disorders,* December 17, 1993; 12: 717–22.

Sanders, L. *The Perfect Fit Diet: Combine What Science Knows About Weight Loss with What You Know About Yourself.* New York: St. Martin's Press, 2004.

Scallet, A. C., and Olney, J. W. Components of hypothalamic obesity: Bipiperidyl-mustard lesions add hyperphagia to monosodium glutamate-induced hyperinsulinemia. *Brain Reseach,* May 28, 1986; 374(2): 380–4.

Scheen, A. J. From obesity to diabetes: why, when and who? *ACTA Clinica Belgica,* 2000; 29(12): 1045–52.

Schmidt, M. A. *Smart Fats.* Berkeley, CA: Frog, Ltd., 1997.

Schwarzbein, D., and Deville, N. *The Schwarzbein Principle: The Truth About Losing Weight, Being Healthy and Feeling Younger.* Deerfield Beach, FL: Health Communications, 1999.

Sears, B. *The Anti-Aging Zone.* New York: HarperCollins, 1999.

Seelig, M. S. Magnesium requirements in human nutrition. *Magnesium Bulletin,* 1981; 3(1A): 26–47.

Sergio, W. A natural food, Malabar Tamarind, may be effective in the treatment of obesity. *Medical Hypotheses,* 1988; 27: 39–40.

Seroy, S. Response to JAMA HCA report. *Townsend Letter for Doctors and Patients,* February/March 1999; 120–1 [letter/review].

Severson, K. *The Trans Fat Solution.* Berkeley, CA: Ten Speed Press, 2003.

Simoneau, J. A., et al. Markers of capacity to utilize fatty acids in human skeletal muscle: Relation to insulin resistance and obesity and effects of weight loss. *FASEB Journal*, 1999; 13(14): 2051–60.

Simopoulos, A. P., and Robinson, J. *The Omega Diet*. New York: HarperCollins Publishers, 1998.

Simson, E. L., Gold, R. M., Standish, L. J., and Pellett, P. L. Axon-sparing brain lesioning technique: The use of monosodium-L-glutamate and other amino acids. *Science*, November 4, 1977; 198(4316): 515–17.

Slyper, A. H. Childhood obesity, adipose tissue distribution and the pediatric practitioner. *Pediatrics*, 1998; 102(1): E4.

Soft Drink Association. *Estimated Annual Production and Consumption of Soft Drinks*. Washington, DC, 1987.

Stein, J. Paging Dr. Fatkins? In the low-carb vs. low-fat war, the Furu's health becomes exhibit A. Did his diet help do him in? *TIME*, February 23, 2004.

Stewart, H. L., et al. *The New Sugar Busters: Cut Sugar to Trim Fat*. New York: Ballantine Books, 2003.

Stoll, A. *The Omega-3 Connection*. London: Simon & Schuster, 2001.

Story, M. School-based approaches for preventing and treating obesity. *International Journal of Obesity Related Metabolic Disorder*, 1999 (supplement), 23: S43–51.

Strand, C. *All About Water: Water Contamination and Its Effect on Our Health*, 2001, pp. 8–10; www.waterwarning.com.

Strauss, R. Childhood obesity. *Current Problems in Pediatrics*, 1999; 29(1): 1–29.

Sullivan, A. C., Hamilton, J. G., Miller, O. N., et al. Inhibition of lipogenesis in rat liver by (-)-hydroxycitrate. *Archives of Biochemistry and Biophysics*, 1972; 150: 183–90.

Sullivan, A. C., and Triscari, J. Metabolic regulation as a control for lipid disorders. *American Journal of Clinical Nutrition*, 1977; 30: 767–76.

Sullivan, A. C., Triscari, J., Hamilton, J. G., et al. Effect of (-)-hydroxycitrate upon the accumulation of lipid in the rat: I. Lipogenesis. *Lipids*, 1974; 9: 121–28.

Sullivan, A. C., Triscari, J., Hamilton, J. G., et al. Effect of (-)-hydroxycitrate upon the accumulation of lipid in the rat: II. Appetite. *Lipids*, 1974; 9: 129–34.

Tanaka, K., Shimada, M., Nakao, K., and Kusunoki, T. Hypothalamic lesion induced by injection of monosodium glutamate in suckling period and subsequent development of obesity. *Experimental Neurology*, October 1978; 62(1): 191–99.

Tarnower, H., and Baker, S. S. *The Complete Scarsdale Medical Diet.* New York: Bantam Books, 1980.

Thom, E., Wadstein, J., and Gudmundsen, O. Conjugated linoleic acid reduces body fat in healthy excercising humans. *International Medical Research*, 2001; 29: 392–96.

Tokuyama, K., and Himms-Hagen, J. Adrenalectomy prevents obesity in glutamate-treated mice. *American Journal of Physiology*, August 1989; 257(2 Pt 1): E139–44.

Triscari, J., and Sullivan, A. C. Comparative effects of (-)-hydroxycitrate and (+)-allo-hydroxycitrate on acetyl CoA-carboxylase and fatty acid and cholesterol synthesis in vivo. *Lipids*, 1977; 12: 357–63.

Udall, K. G. *Flaxseed Oil: The Premiere Source of Omega-3 Fatty Acids.* Pleasant Grove, UT: Woodland Publishing, 1997.

Vale, J. *Chocolate Busters: The Easy Way to Kick It!* London: Thorsons, Hammersmith, 2004.

van Dale, D., et al. Weight maintenance and resting metabolic rate 18–40 months after a diet/exercise treatment. *International Journal of Obesity*, April 1990; 14(4): 347–59.

Vincent, J. B. Mechanisms of chromium action: Low-molecular-weight chromium-binding substance. *Journal of the American College of Nutrition*, 1999; 18(1): 6–12.

Walker, M. *Jumping for Health: A Guide to Rebounding Aerobics.* Garden City Park, NY: Avery Publishing Group, 1989, pp. 11, 42–45, 60, and 62.

Walker, M. Phytochemicals in soybeans. *Health Foods Business*, March 1995; 36.

Warren, R. *The Purpose Driven Life.* Grand Rapids, MI: Zondervan, 2002.

Junk food and school lunches. *Well Being Journal,* May/June 2004; 13(3): 1.

Westerterp, K. R., et al. Diet induced thermogenesis measured over 24th in a respiration chamber: Effect of diet composition. *International Journal of Obesity and Related Metabolic Disorders*, 1999; 23(3): 287–92.

Wilcox, B., and Wilcox, D. C. *The Okinawa Program: Learn the Secrets to Healthy Longevity.* New York: Three Rivers Press, 2001.

Willet, W. C., et al. Is dietary fat a major determinant of body fat? *American Journal of Clinical Nutrition*, 1998; 67: 556S–562S.

Wills, J. *The Omega Diet: A Revolutionary Approach to LifeLong Weight Loss and Wellbeing.* London: Headline Publishing, 2001.

Wurtman, R. J., and Lewis, M. C. Exercise, plasma composition and neurotransmission. In *Advances in Nutrition and Top Sport* (vol. 32), ed. F. Brouns. Basel: Karger, 1991, pp. 94–109.

Wyatt, C., et al. Dietary intake of sodium, potassium, and blood pressure in lacto-ovo vegetarians. *Nutrition Research*, 1995; 15: 819–30.

Yanick, P., Jr., Ph.D., and Haffee, R., M.D., Ph.D. *Clinical Chemistry and Nutrition: A Physicians Desk Reference*. Lake Ariel, PA: T & H Publishing.

Yoshioka, K., Yoshida, T., and Kondo, M. Reduced brown adipose tissue thermogenesis and metabolic rate in pre-obese mice treated with monosodium-L-glutamate. *Endocrinologia Japonica*, February 1991; 38(1): 75–79.

Young, R. *Herbal Nutritional Medications*. Alpine, UT: Hikari Holdings Publishing, 1988.

Young, R. *Sick and Tired*. Lindon, UT: Woodland Publishing, 2000.

Young, R., and Young, S. *The pH Miracle*. New York: Warner Books, 2002.

Young, R., and Young, S. *The pH Miracle for Diabetes*. New York: Warner Books, 2004.

Young, R., and Young, S. *Why Drink SuperGreens*. Orem, UT: Sounds Concepts Publishing, 2003.

Young, S. *Back to the House of Health*. Lindon, UT: Woodland Publishing, 1999.

Young, S. *Back to the House of Health II*. Lindon, UT: Woodland Publishing, 2003.

Yudkin, J. Evolutionary and historical changes in dietary carbohydrates. *American Journal of Clinical Nutrition*, 1967; 20(2): 108–15.

Zimmerman, M. *Eat Your Colours: Maximize Your Health by Eating the Right Foods for Your Body Type*. London: Metro Publishing, 2002.

Zoltan, P. R., *Return to the Joy of Health: Natural Medicine and Alternative Treatment for All Your Health Complaints*. Vancouver: Alive Books, 1995.

Zorad, S., Macho, L., Jezova, D., and Fickova, M. Partial characterization of insulin resistance in adipose tissue of monosodium glutamate-induced obese rats. *Annals of the New York Academy of Science*, September 20, 1997; 827: 541–45.

Index

Page numbers of illustrations appear in italics.

About the Authors

ROBERT O. YOUNG, PH.D., D.SC., is a nationally reowned microbiologist and nutritionist who speaks to audiences around the world on health and wellness. He holds a degree in microbiology and nutrition and has devoted his life to researching the cause of disease and helping people reclaim their health and well-being. Dr. Young is head of the pH Miracle Living Foundation and has gained national recognition for his research into diabetes, cancer, leukemia, and AIDS. He is a member of the American Society of Microbiologists and the American Naturopathic Association and conducts classes in live blood analysis and the "New Biology."

SHELLEY REDFORD YOUNG, L.M.T., is a licensed massage therapist with a passionate interest in optimum nutrition. With Dr. Young she speaks to audiences around the world on the basic requirements of a healthful diet, sharing her delicious, alkalizing, vegetarian recipes (many examples giving in this book).

Together, Robert and Shelley Young provide a dynamic dose of helath and nutrition expertise, guaranteed to inform and en*light*en. They are the authors of *The pH Miracle* and *The pH Miracle for Diabetes*.